PEDIATRIC PHYSICAL THERAPY STRENGTHENING EXERCISES FOR THE KNEES

PEDIATRIC PHYSICAL THERAPY STRENGTHENING EXERCISES FOR THE KNEES

*Treatment Suggestions
by
Muscle Action*

Amy E. Sturkey, PT

Pediatric Physical Therapy Strengthening Exercises for the Knees
Copyright © 2020 by Amy E. Sturkey, PT

All rights reserved. Printed in the United States of America. This book may be used or reproduced for client or therapist education without prior written permission from the author, for non-monetary gain, as long as credit is provided to the author.

For information contact:
Amy E. Sturkey, PT
amysturkey@gmail.com
www.igotchaapps.com

Book and Cover design by Guy Bryant

ISBN: 978-0-9981567-6-7
First Edition: May 2020

DEDICATION

This book is dedicated to all PT students who asked for treatment ideas and every mother who wanted help for her child.

CONTENTS

I. KNEE EXTENSION..1

II. KNEE FLEXION..71

III. ABOUT THE THE AUTHOR..........................106

IV. OTHER OFFERINGS BY AUTHOR............ 107

I. KNEE EXTENSION

THE KNEE EXTENSORS INCREASE THE angle between the femur and tibia. The ankle moves further from the buttock. This movement is in the sagittal plane. The knee extensors are critical for everyday movements like walking, running, jumping, and moving from sitting to standing. Weakness or tightness in the knee extensors will affect functional mobility and is a key component in crouch walking. This chapter includes a wide variety of exercises to improve knee extensor strength.

* * *

1. HIP/KNEE EXTENSION SUPINE ON BALL

I tend to use this exercise with clients who have little idea or capability of pushing with hip and knee extension. If you carefully balance the client on the ball, then a small hip/knee extension push from the client produces a big and rewarding movement. I often end up taking this kind of client through the movement so she can get the feel of the motion. Usually, the client will be motivated by the action and want to repeat it. The further you have the client on top of the ball, the more gravity-eliminated this movement becomes.

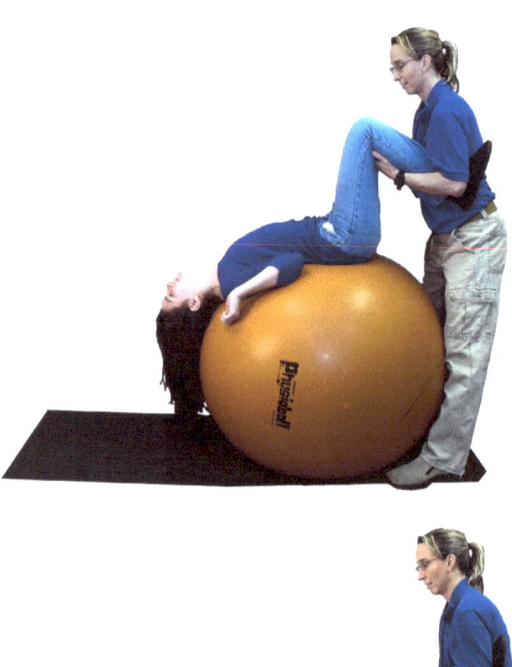

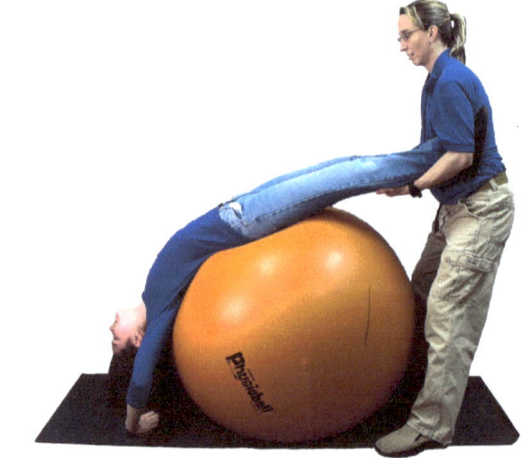

PEDIATRIC PHYSICAL THERAPY STRENGTHENING EXERCISES FOR THE KNEES

2. BILATERAL KNEE/HIP EXTENSION WITH A SCOOTERBOARD

Really, any easily rolled object will do. You can use a skateboard, a toy car, sliding disk, or a bolster under the child's legs. I bend the child's legs up, and then he pushes them out. Sometimes I put blocks out at the end range for the child to knock down at the end of the movement. Kids love knocking things down.

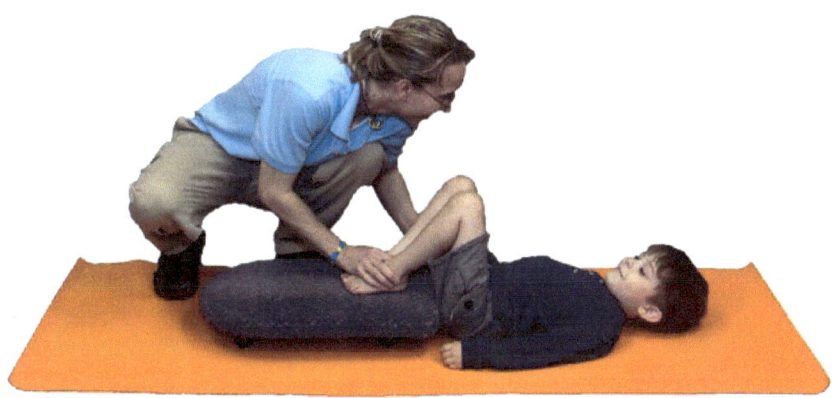

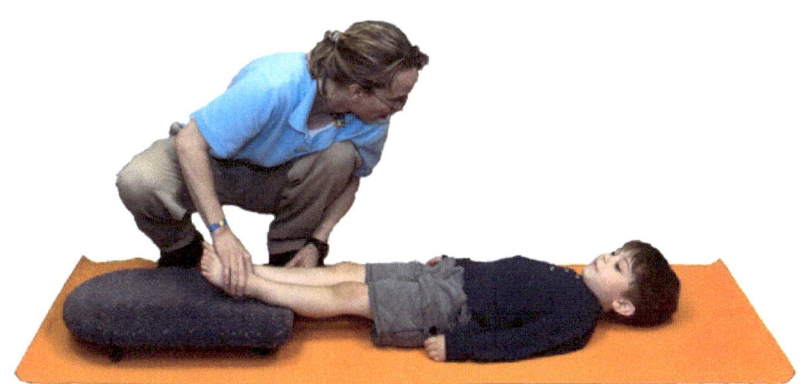

3. SUPINE BICYCLE

This exercise works bilateral alternating hip and knee extension (and flexion.) If this is too hard, try reverting to both legs flexing and extending. Some children may not be able to motor plan alternating the flexion and extension.

I use this exercise with manual assistance when my client is clueless about how to perform the movement. I use elastic bands or manual resistance when a child has more strength and a high level of cooperation. I have found this is a particularly excellent exercise after the Selective Dorsal Rhizotomy. Pelvic disassociation is always tricky for my clients with quadriplegic or diplegic cerebral palsy. This activity is a wonderful way to encourage moving one leg significantly different than the other. This exercise technically works knee/hip flexion on one leg with knee/hip extension on the other leg, reciprocally and alternating.

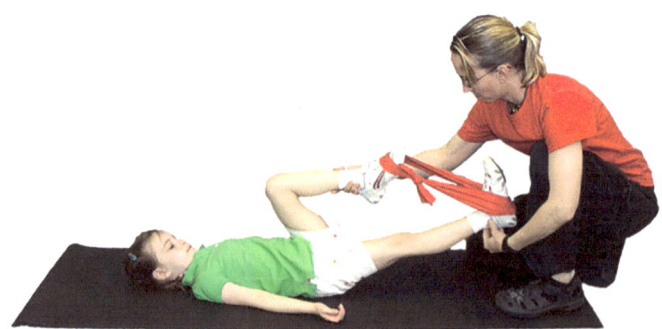

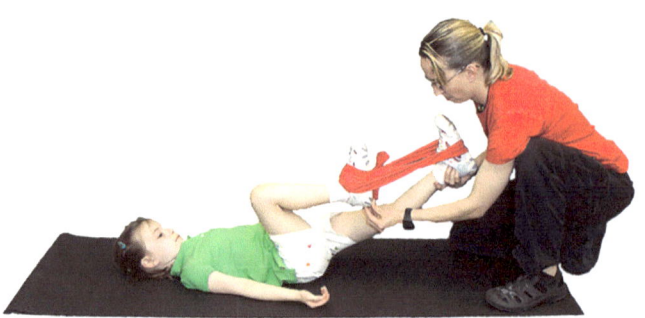

4. QUAD SETS

I don't usually employ this classic quad strengthening exercise. I have plenty of children who need terminal knee extension. I think I strongly prefer closed chain exercises. When I do this exercise, I try to find something that makes a sound when pressed to go under the knees. I typically use dog squeak toys. I have some that squeak easily and some that are quite hard to squeak. The louder the noise is, the better the reward. I also may just put my hand under the child's knee and push up against them to make this more challenging. I make it a competition saying, "I can make you bend your knee." I get to try until I count to 10. My kids ALWAYS love beating me.

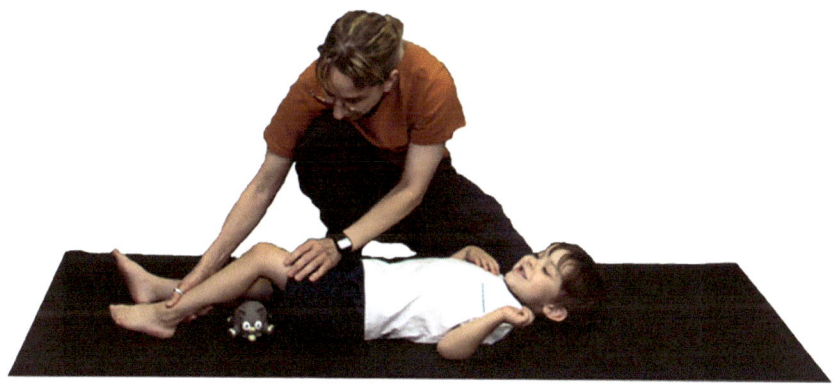

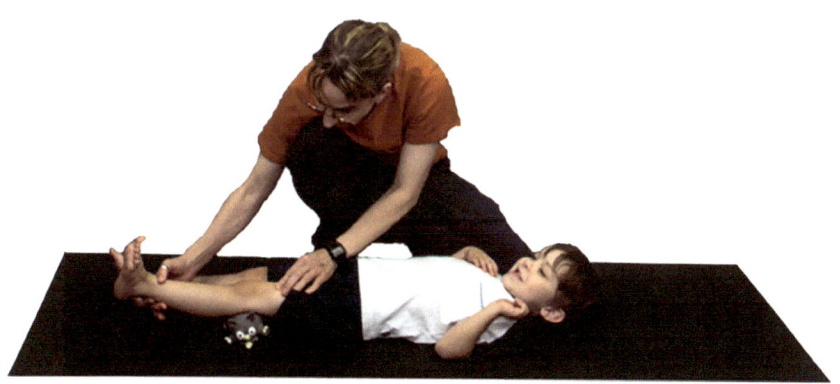

5. SHORT ARC QUADS

Another classic quad strengthening exercise that I rarely do. I probably should. Perform this exercise for repetitions with and without ankle weights. At the clinic, we have soft velcro ankle weights ranging from ¼ lb to 3 lbs. Something like, "I bet you can't lift this weight to my hand" usually works. If he is successful with one weight, I add more until I have found the perfect weight.

In the picture, my model had to extend his knee to lift his foot to touch the car he wanted. After 10 reps, he put ten cars down a ramp. I also have the child extend his knee and hold it for 10 seconds. Or I do the eccentric version in which I claim I can push his foot back down to the floor within 10 seconds. Beating me in a competition is always a winning game for both of us.

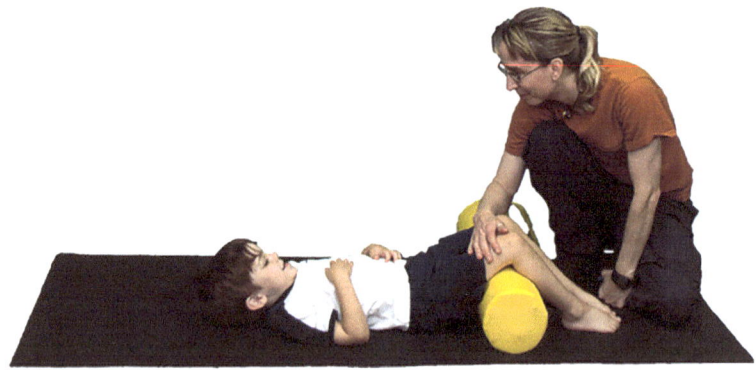

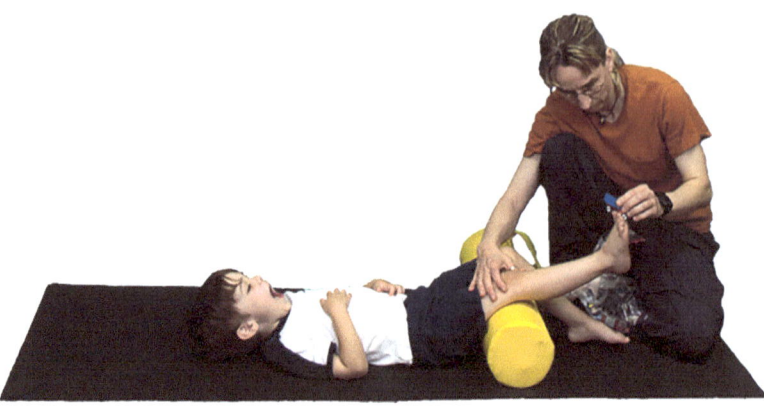

6. STRAIGHT LEG RAISE

I guess I'll get the classic exercises listed first. Again, I can't tell you the last time I did this exercise. I do this most frequently with my post-rhizotomy clients who aren't walking yet. I emphasize getting terminal knee extension first before lifting the leg. I only go as high as the client can go and keep the full knee extension. You could encourage a little self-competition. "Let's see how many repetitions you can get in 30 seconds." Or you could use weights on their thigh or ankle and see what the child's skill is. I perform this exercise, concentrically, eccentrically, or isometrically, with resistance by hand or from Velcro weights.

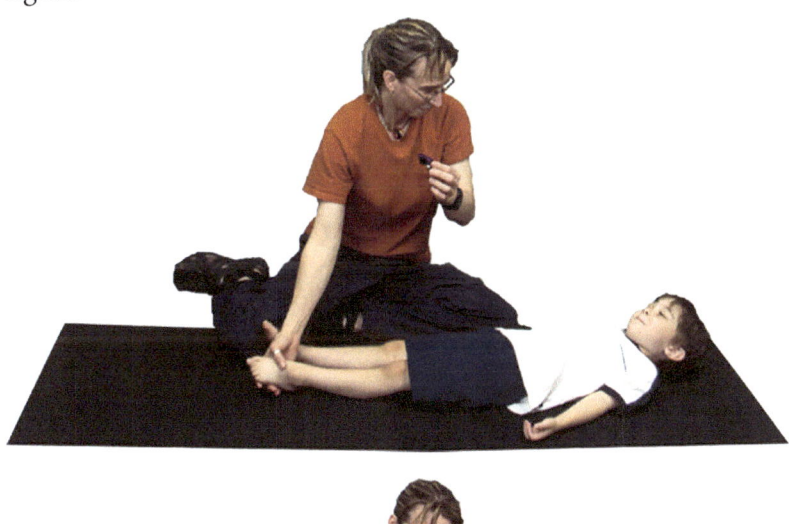

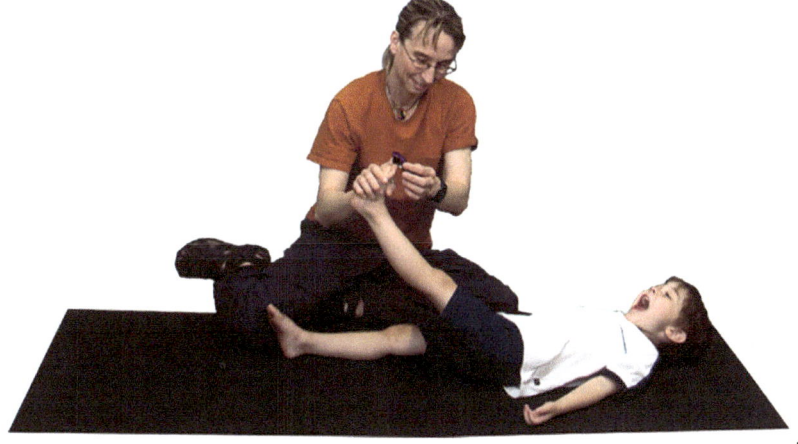

7. SWING SEATED PRESS

This activity is a much more enjoyable way to practice knee extension. I use the platform swing since it has a little more weight on it. For some children, I am merely trying to get them to use knee extension to get the swing to go. For others, I have the child push and hold knee extension to hold the swing back from the neutral hanging down position for a specified amount of time. The leg press is harder if I am on the swing behind them, adding the extra weight.

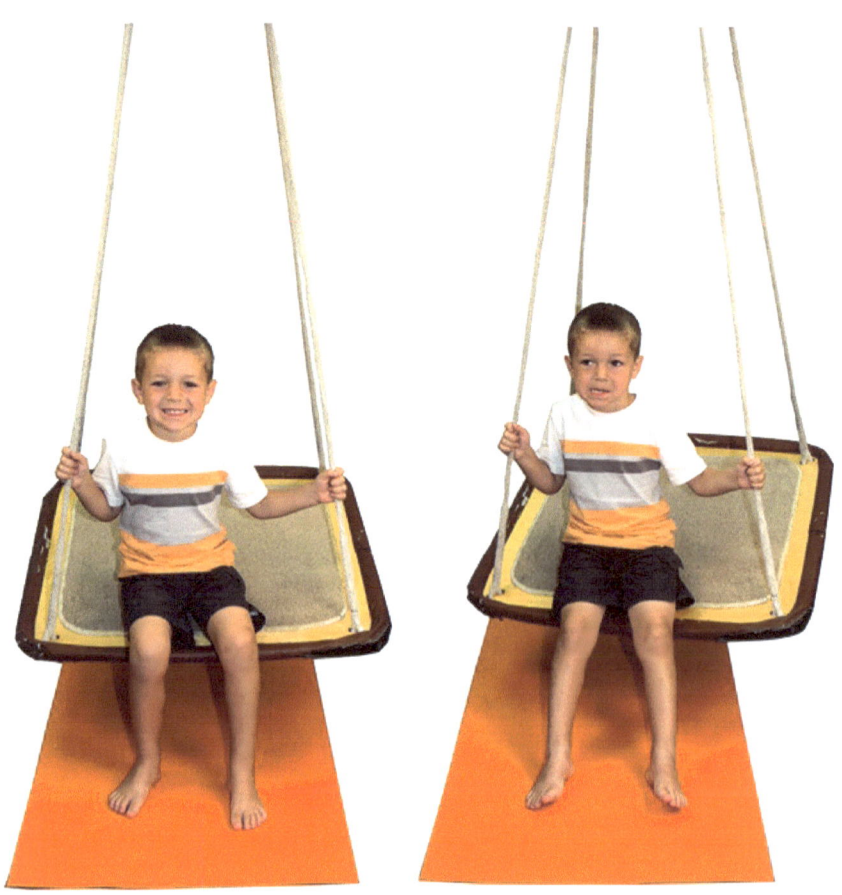

8. TWO LEGS HIP/KNEE EXTENSION, SUPINE

Ah, the human squat press machine! I use this exercise frequently. Kids love this activity. I put the child lying back on a bean bag or pillow blocked behind by a wall or large furniture. This prevents the child from sliding away from me on the floor. I often have a parent stabilize his shoulders to keep him from moving. I help the child flex his hips and knees to end range. Then I lean forward, putting my upper chest on the child's feet. I adjust my weight on the child applying just enough pressure for the child to just barely be successful in pushing me off. I fall dramatically. Oh, the kids love this exercise. I have no problems getting 8-10 repetitions. I have used this with clients who are minimally or severely physically involved. It works perfectly.

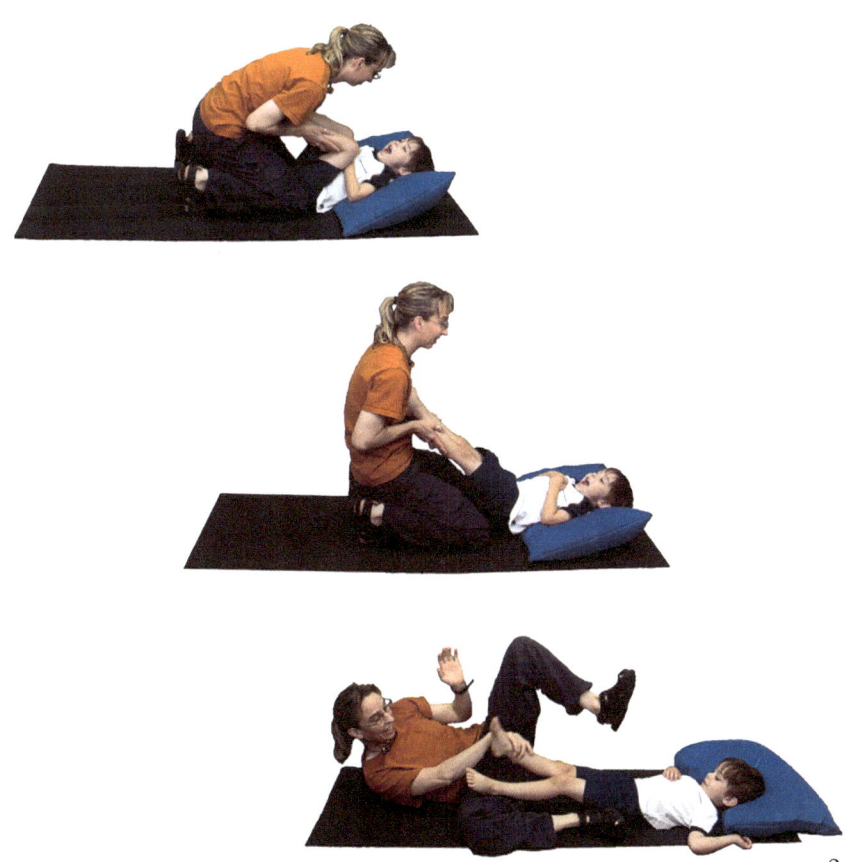

9. ONE LEG HIP/KNEE EXTENSION, SUPINE

I should have called this the one-legged squat press machine! I use this activity when I want to isolate one leg at a time. It is excellent for children with one-sided involvement. Kids still love this activity. Using the same set up as the previous activity, I help the child flex his hip and knee to end range. I block the other leg down relatively straight. The child typically begs for more.

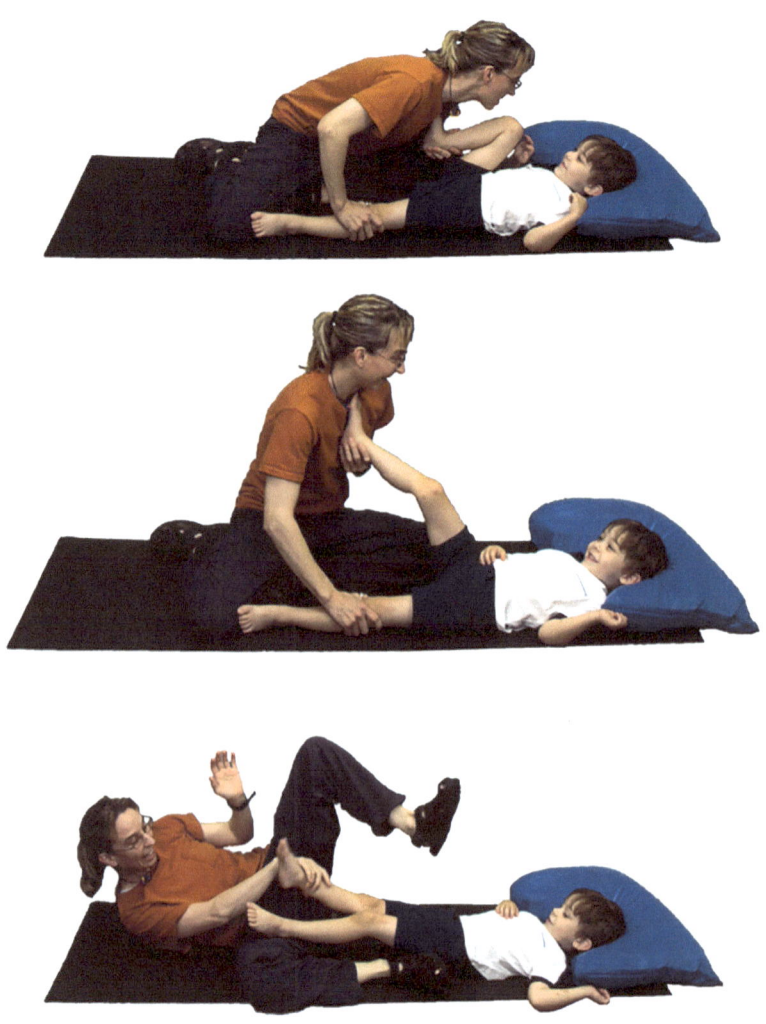

10. LEG PRESS WITH THERABAND

Here is a variation of the leg press in which the child holds the theraband and performs the leg press by herself. Of course, this requires a motivated and cooperative client. I strongly recommend theraband over theratubing for this activity. Theratubing tends to roll and snap back on the child.

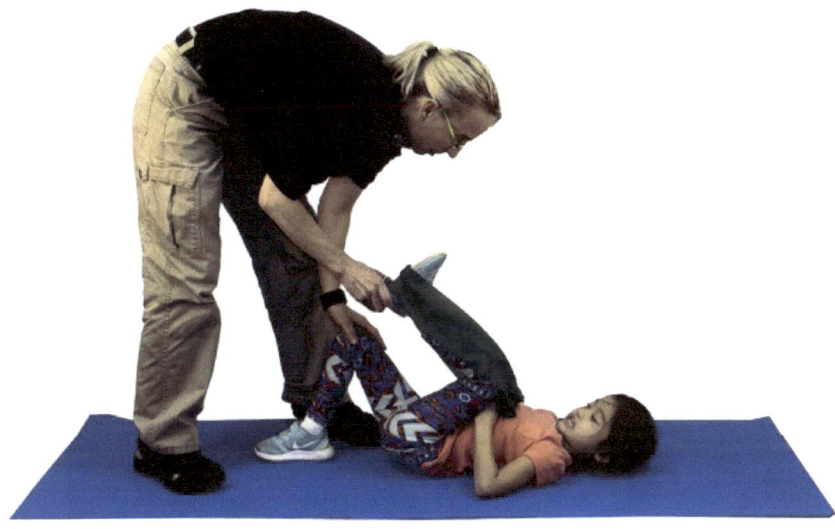

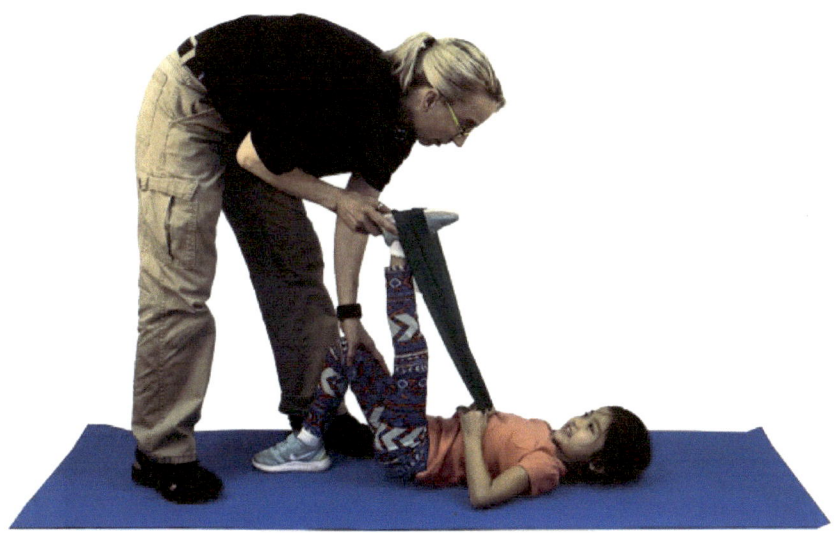

11. SEATED RESISTED KNEE EXTENSION

Concentrically, I start with the child in knee flexion, and I resist the child fully extending the knee. I put the closer of my wrists under the back of the child's knee and then apply resistance at his shin with my free hand (not as pictured). I put my nose at the end range position for the child's foot. I count slowly to 5, and I taunt the child, "I bet you can't lift your foot to my nose!" I resist just enough that the child barely makes it to my nose by the count of 5. When he does, I complain at how awful his stinky socks smell. Kids love this.

To perform this eccentrically, I need a target like a block placed at end range knee flexion (or at 90 degrees knee flexion as I typically do.) I use the same taunt technique, but it is never quite as fun because my nose is not at the end. I challenge the child to keep his foot/heel from knocking over the block. "I am going to try to make you knock that block down. You push really hard and try to stop me." And then the battle is on. Again I push just hard enough that the child almost, but doesn't, knock down the block by the count of 5 or 10. You could do similarly isometrically and taunt the child that he can't keep his foot on your nose. Anyway I do this; kids love to beat the therapist.

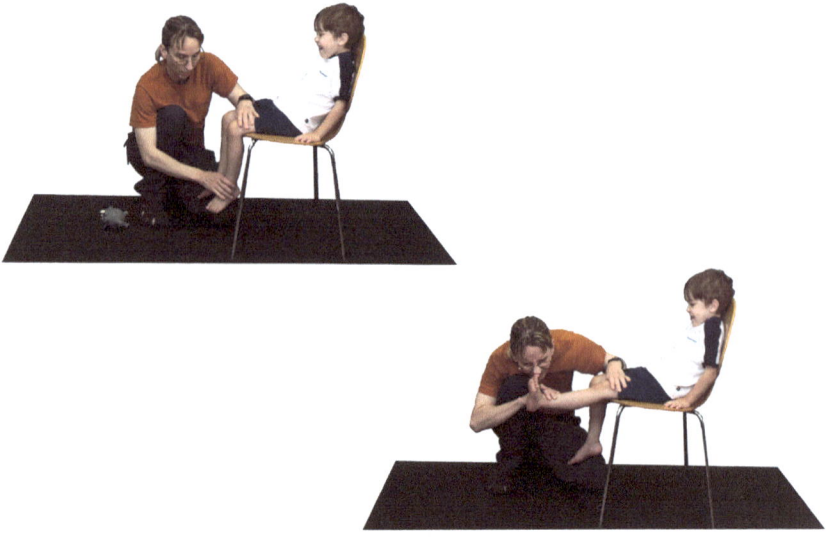

12. SEATED SCOOTERBOARD PUSH

Sometimes I have to block the child's feet or help the child keep his heels down on the ground. If the child is more capable, then I race the child down the hall. I ride on my scooterboard, and the race is on! If the child is quite strong, I have him alternate pushing with one foot and then the other, instead of two at a time. I always do this exercise on hard floor, such as the vinyl tile that we have at the clinic. The resistance on the carpet would be tough to overcome.

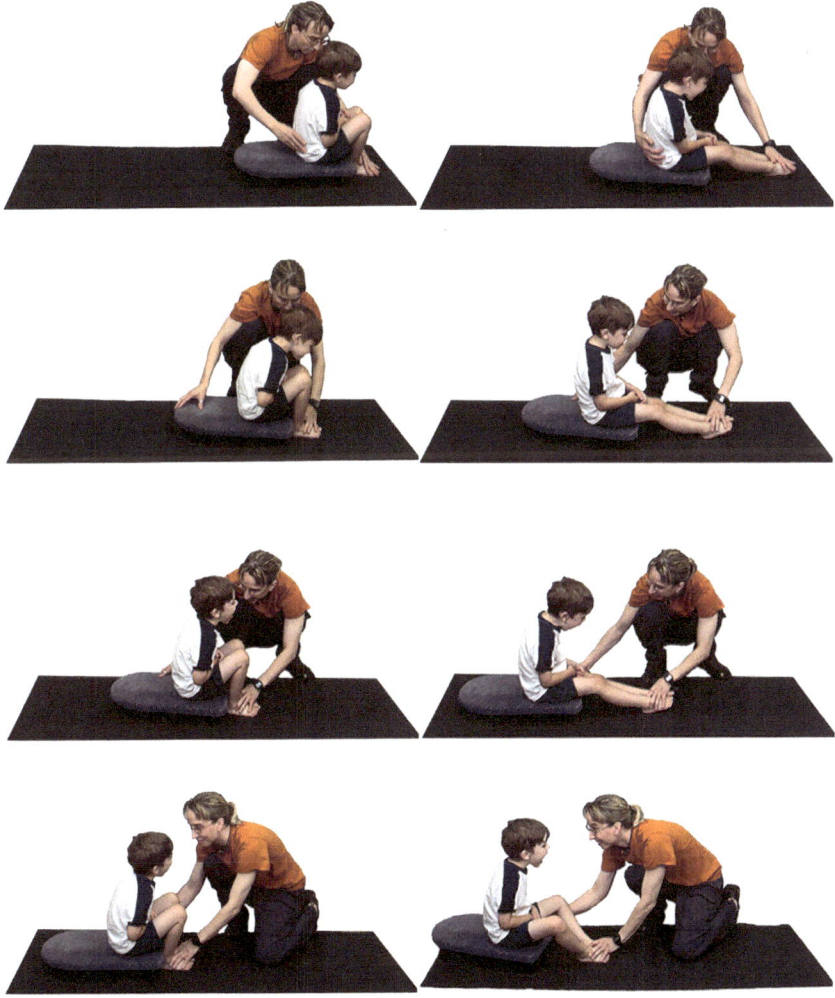

13. SEATED SCOOTERBOARD PUSH, ONE LEG AT A TIME

Want twice the work? Instead of two legs, only allow the child to push with one leg at a time, with or without assistance.

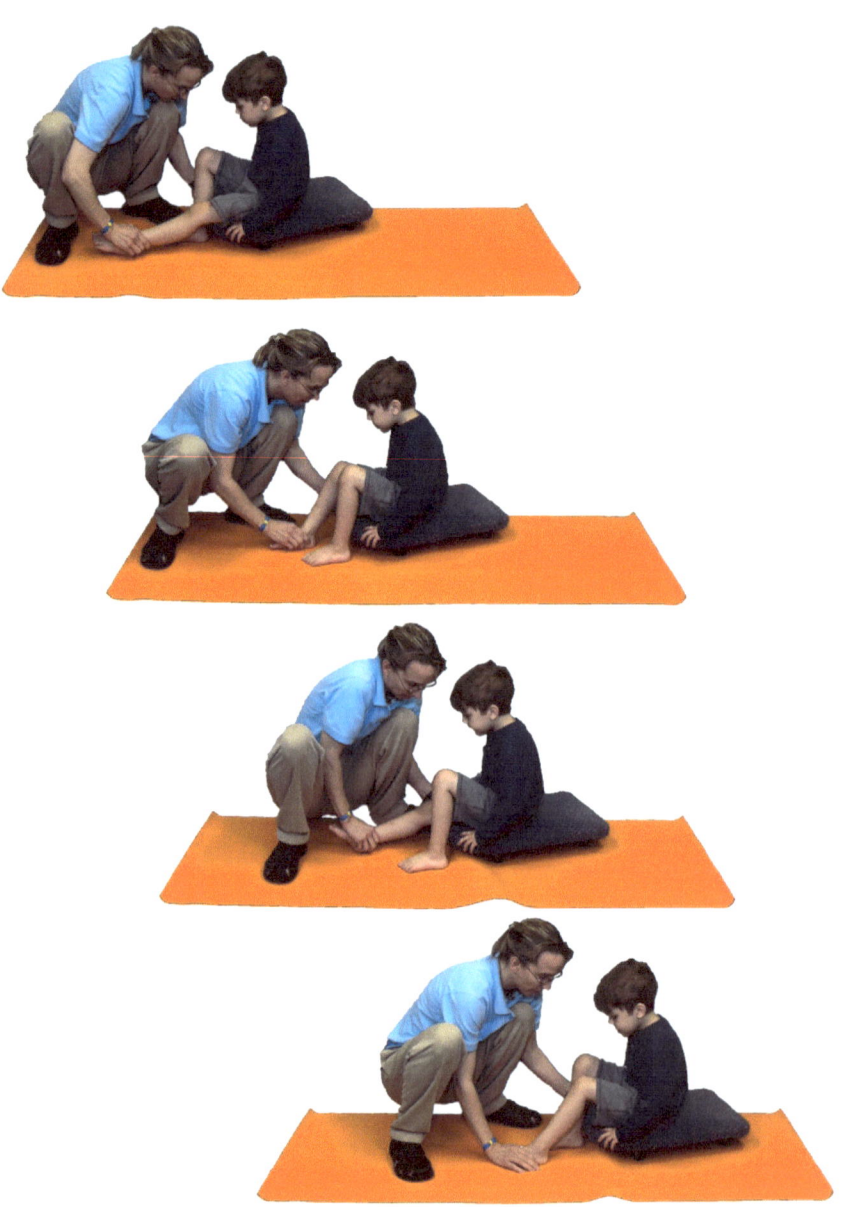

14. BOUNCING SITTING ON A BALL

This is a straightforward exercise. Sometimes I stabilize the ball as seen in this photo, and sometimes I can sit beside the child and bounce as well. I usually bring a ball for the parent and make a party out of it. I always put down the mat if I am worried that the child might fall. The higher you have the child bounce and the lower the ball, the harder this activity is. I tend to get a ball that is the height of the back of the child's knee when the child is sitting on it. This activity is a deceiving activity. I often end up sitting on a small ball myself, and my quads fatigue while doing this activity.

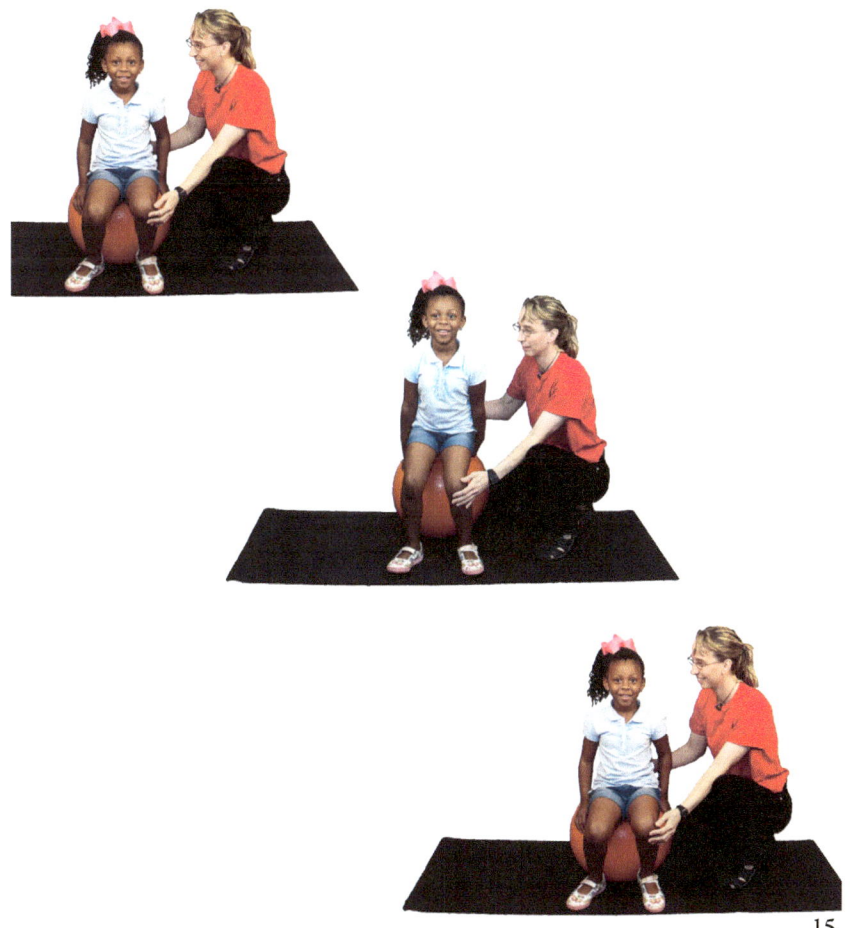

15. HIGH FRONT KNEE KICK

I usually do this game with a tetherball, but any target will do. I ask my child to keep her leg cocked up, and as the tetherball swings to her, she kicks it. If a client can't keep her leg up in hip flexion, I allow the child to put her leg down on the floor between each repetition. The higher the tetherball/target, the harder this is. When using a tetherball, I like to have the parent help me. I have the parent stand on one end of the arc of the tetherball, and the client and I stand at the other end of the arc. I have the mother hold the tetherball with the rope pulled taut between repetitions and release it on cue. In this manner, the arc of the tetherball swing is more regular, and the exercise seems to go more smoothly.

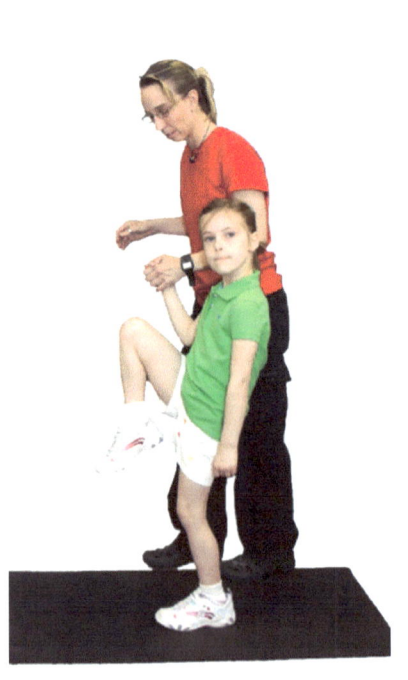
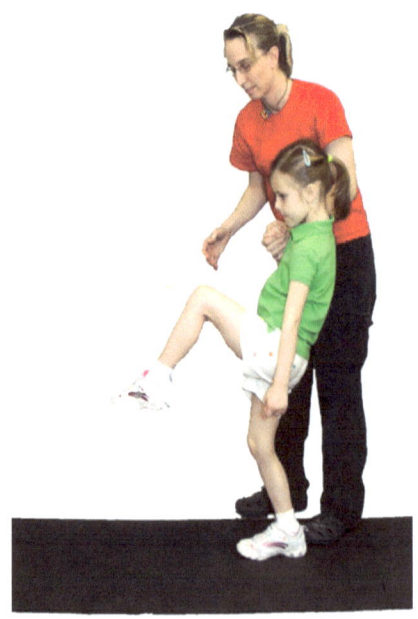

PEDIATRIC PHYSICAL THERAPY STRENGTHENING EXERCISES FOR THE KNEES

16. STRADDLE SIT TO STAND

I have several kids who pull in their adductors as they move from sitting to standing. Straddling something like a bench or a bolster makes adduction a little easier to block. Usually I have to sit behind the client on the bolster and help keep the knees apart with my hands on their knees.

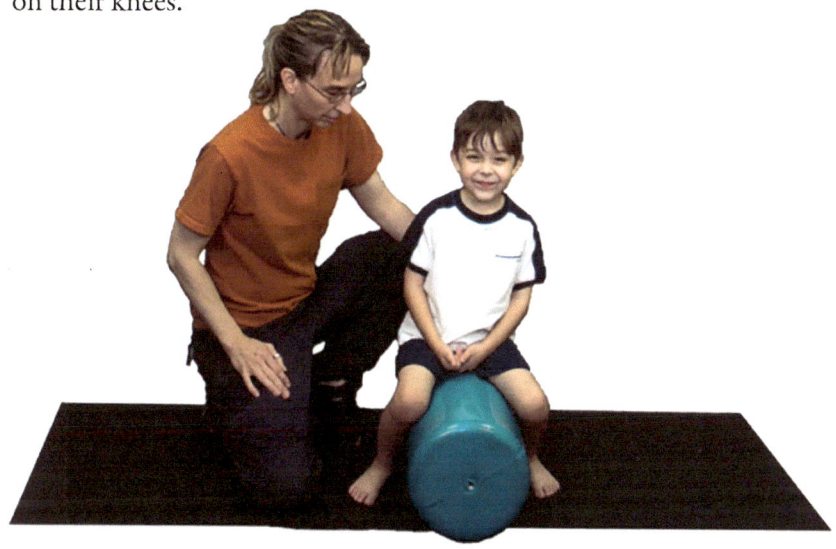

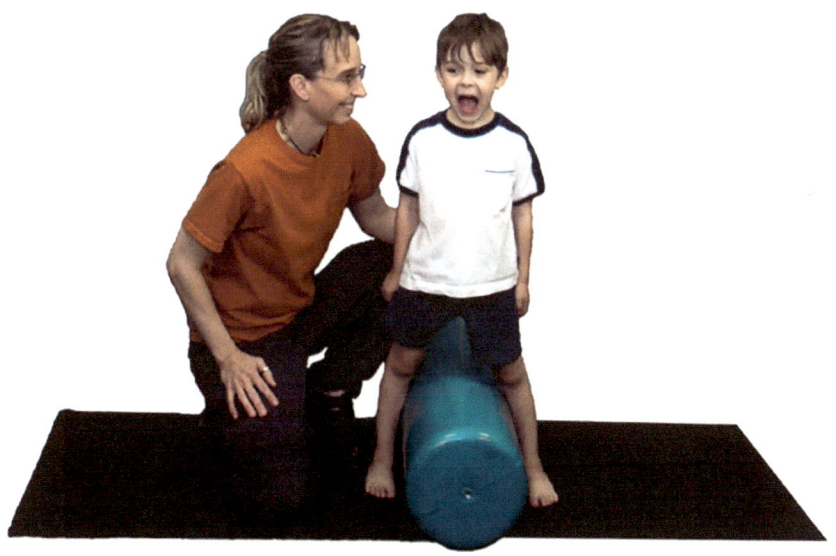

17. SIT TO STAND

Sit to stand is such a functional daily life skill. To give the most support, I use two Kaye Products upright poles, two wall grips, or two hands held. I have suction cup-wall grips meant for showers. I place them on my mirror in my room. I love them! I can put them where I need-up/down, wider/narrower, or vertical/angled/horizontal. If I am using the poles or the wall grips, I sit behind the client, helping at his hips or knees.

From here, I proceed to one hand held or two hands on a wall. Then I progress to touch or to no support in the transition from sitting to standing. I pay attention to whether or not the client needs back of knee support by the chair. Some clients can only get up to standing independently if the back of their knees hit the chair. I also like to work on sit to stand when the client is close to being independent by helping only at the knees in the front. I sit on a lower bench in front of the client facing him. I have my hands on his knees, helping the weight shift forward for the transition and then aiding his standing balance.

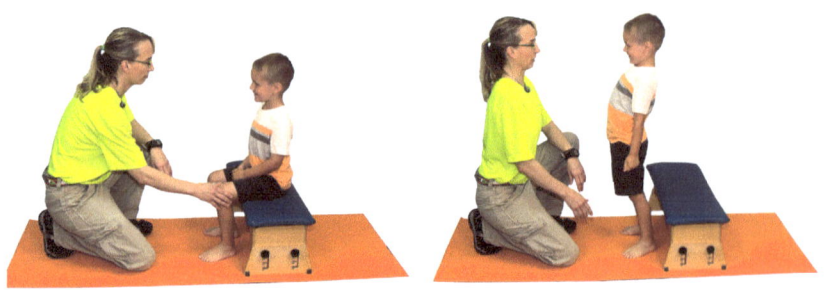

18. LOW BENCH SIT TO STAND

This activity is more challenging with a lower bench. I follow the same progression as described in the previous exercise. You can also emphasize controlling the descent from standing to sitting with control. Sometimes I will ask the child to take up to 10 seconds to sit down. Every inch lower can be much harder for a child, so grade it carefully.

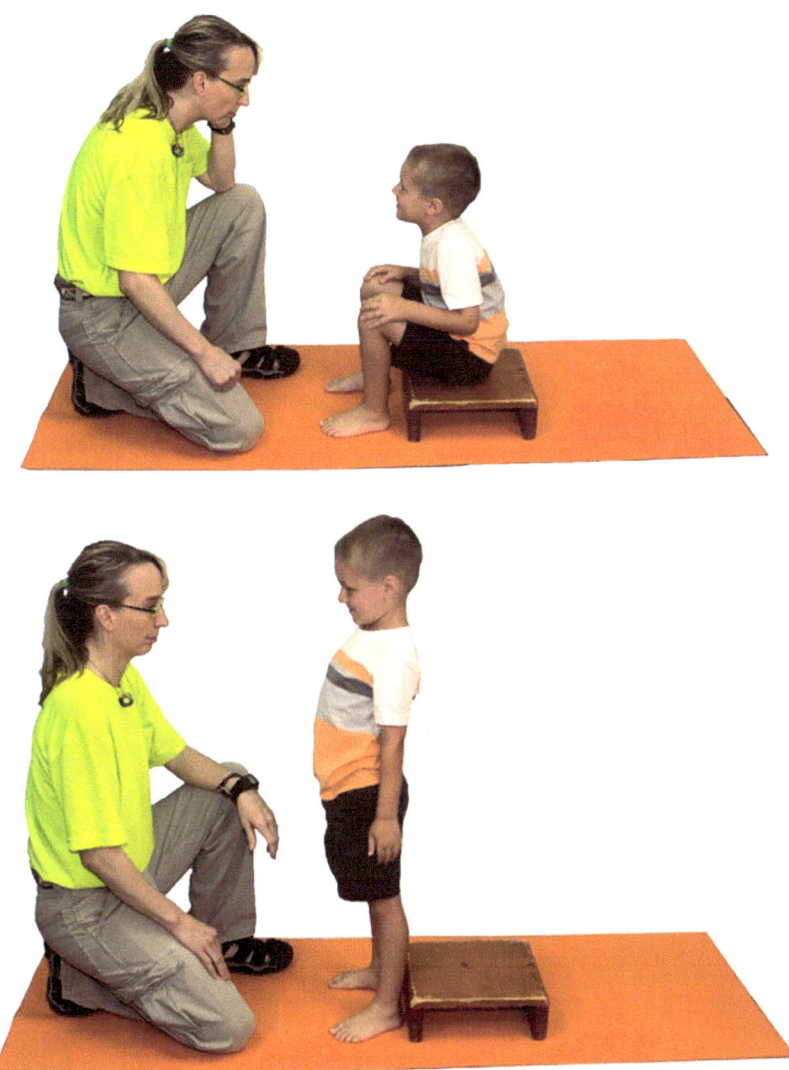

19. TALL BENCH SIT TO STAND

I wouldn't include this, but the higher bench option is so important. I have several more significantly involved children who learned how to perform sit-to-stand or stand-to-sit transfers only from a bench that was much higher than the standard back-of-knee-height. If the child is successful at the tall bench, then you can work lower. If the transfer is going to be difficult for your client, don't start hard, start easy.

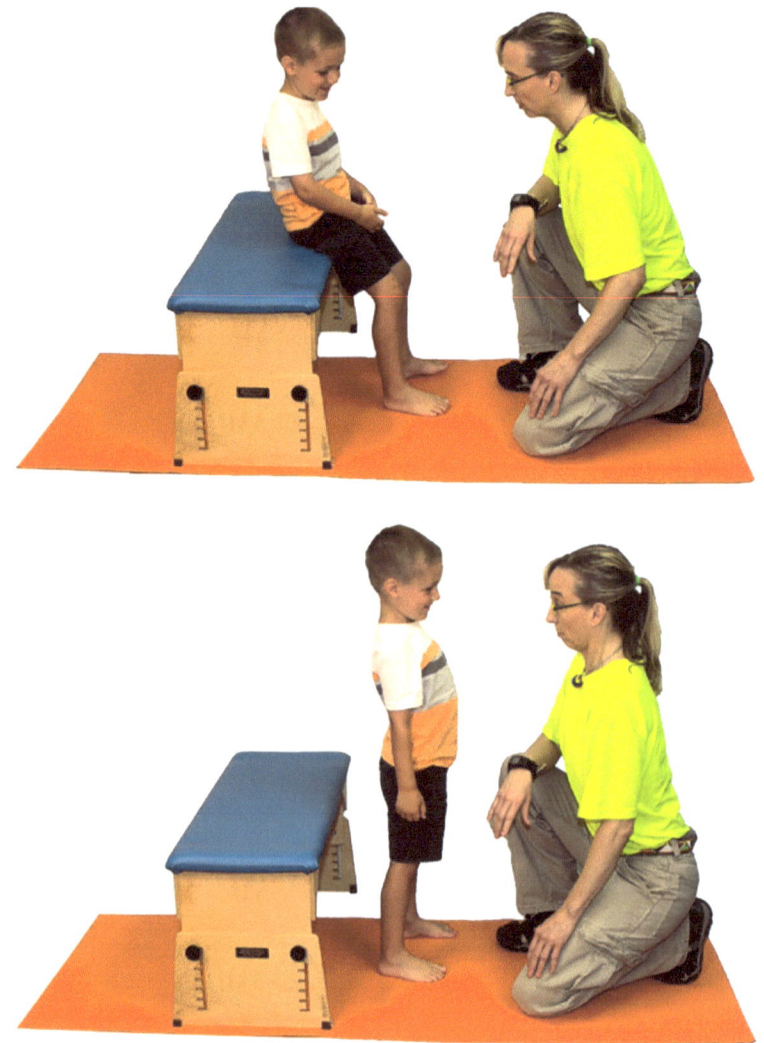

20. TALL BENCH-DON'T SQUEAK!

I have many clients who need to work on midrange control of knee extension. If his hips or knees bend too much, then he collapses down. I love this exercise for midrange control of the knee and hip extensors. I have the client stand in front of a bench with a squeak toy or piano on it. He is to stoop down and touch the piano or squeak toy, but not play/squeak it. This movement is much easier if you don't have to go down too low.

I love the Kaye Products adjustable benches that allow you to modify the benches height one inch at a time until you find the right height for the perfect challenge for the client. If you don't have an adjustable height bench, you can always make the bench effectively an inch shorter by putting a single thickness mat under the client's feet but not under the bench. You can continue along the same lines by doubling and then tripling the mat to make the bench shorter by comparison. I love sound effects, and so do my clients. This exercise is usually fun. Placing the client facing toward a wall mirror helps give him visual feedback about the distance to the squeak toy.

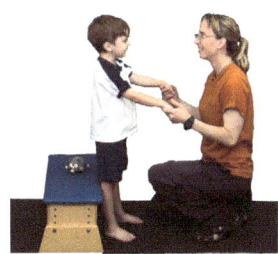 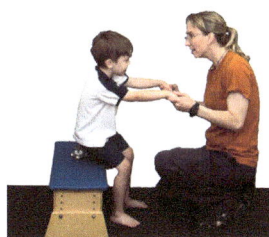 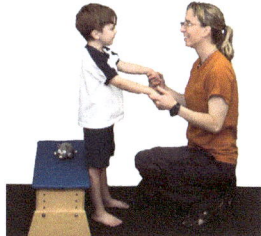

21. LOW BENCH-DON'T SQUEAK!

This is the same as the previous exercise, but one step harder. Simply modifying the bench height even by a small amount can dramatically increase the difficulty.

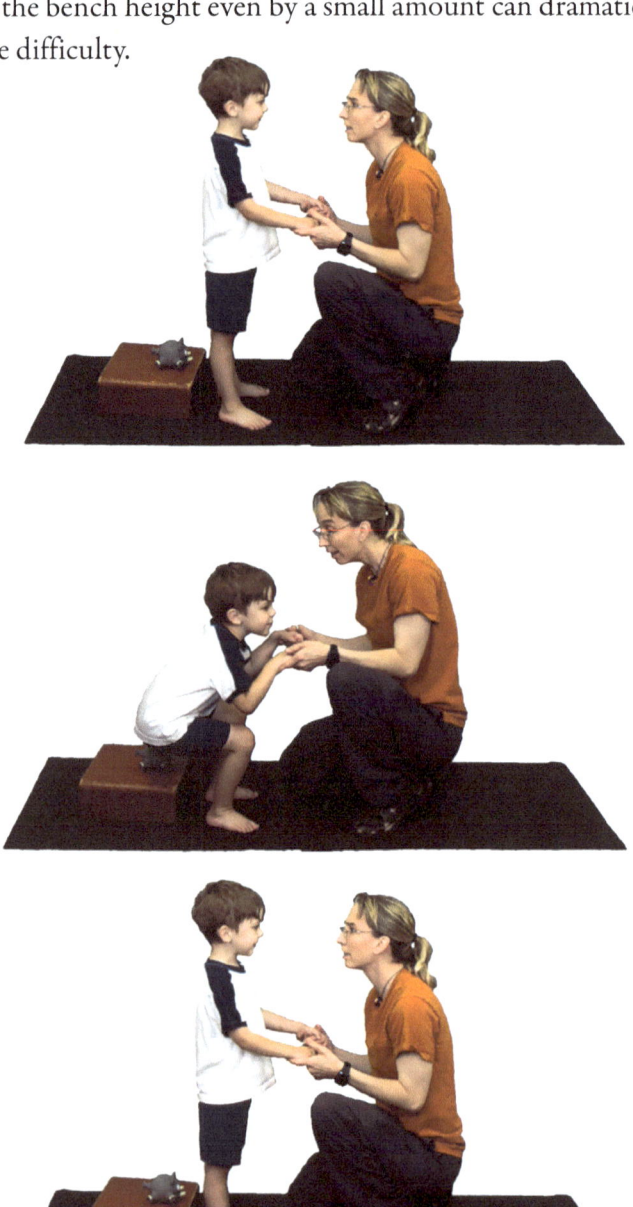

22. SQUAT TO STAND

Squat to stand works hip extensors, quadriceps and plantarflexors, concentrically on the way up and eccentrically on the way down. I try to get children to look up as they transition up and down to try to keep an arch in the back. I try to get my clients to put their heels down. If she has trouble, stand her on a decline or with her heels on a mat and her toes on the floor. Sometimes I assist with one or two hands held. Sometimes I support at the knees from the front. Sometimes I help by sitting on a bench behind her, holding the knees from the back.

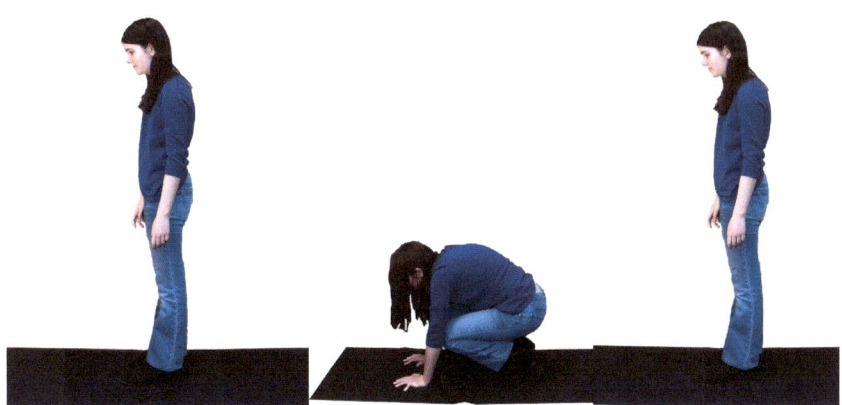

23. LOW TO TALL HALF KNEEL

I usually perform this activity with the child facing a bench. I have the child pick up something on the floor on the side with the knee down. The child has to go down and back to get the puzzle piece, and then he raises into half kneel to put the puzzle piece in the puzzle on the bench. Kids with diplegia find this exercise very difficult. I often have to get in low kneel behind my clients with my knees on either side of the client's further back foot. This gives them the balance needed to perform this activity, especially without a bench. Get rid of the bench for a significantly greater challenge. The quadriceps muscle works concentrically on the way up and eccentrically on the way down.

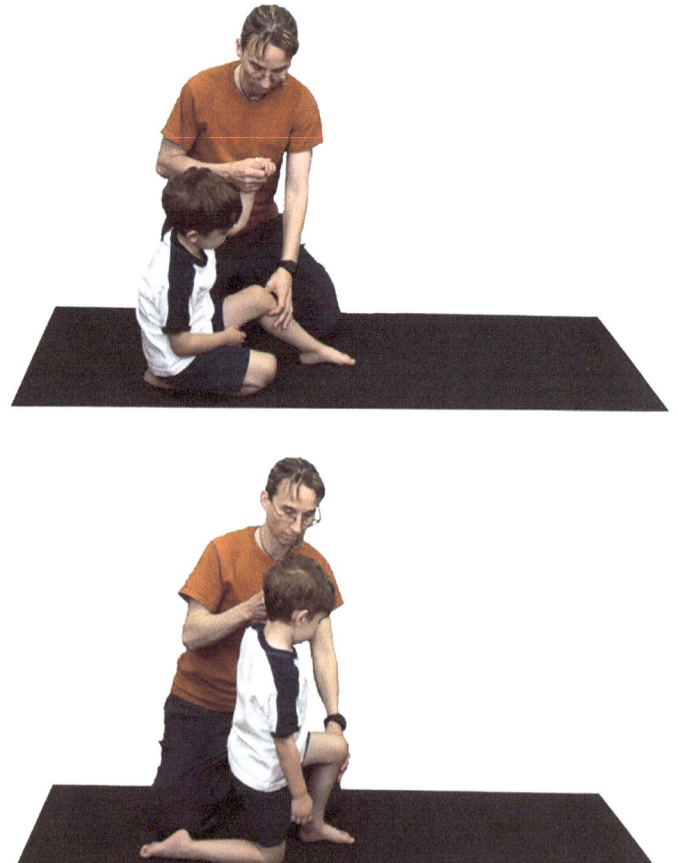

24. HALF KNEEL TO STAND

Half kneel to stand is a terrific hip and knee extension exercise. I work on kneel to half kneel to stand at furniture, at a wall, at two poles, with one pole, with one hand held, or with one hand on the wall with my client facing sideways to the wall. It is important to get the weight shifted forward so that the head is over the knee that is up. Often, I facilitate this transition with knee support from the front when a client is close to independent. Several of my kids have learned to do this movement with both hands on the raised knee. Then I fade to only one hand allowed on the raised knee and then entirely independently. I am not typically satisfied until a child can perform 5-10 repetitions with either leg raised and with hands-free for the transition up and back down again.

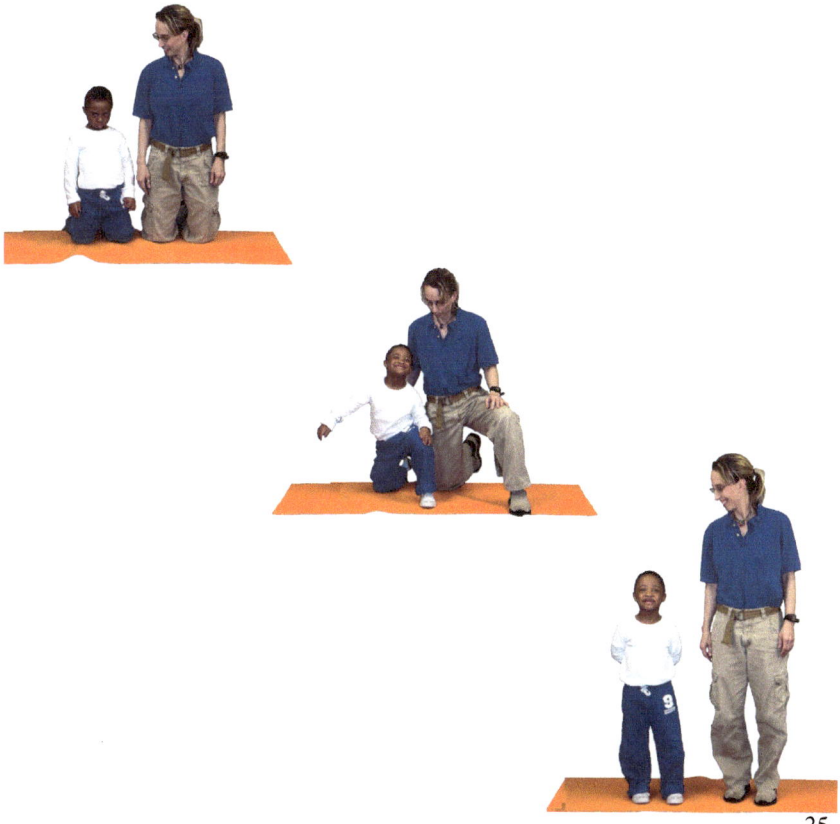

25. STAND TO HALF KNEEL

I also emphasize the transition from standing to half kneel. Most of my clients figure out the transition into standing with control before they can control standing to half kneel. I frequently have to be behind them to guide the back leg down and posteriorly for them to initiate the transition. The movement up to standing emphasizes the concentric muscle contraction. Controlling the descent works the same muscle groups eccentrically.

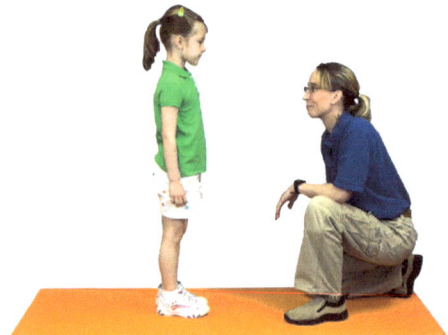

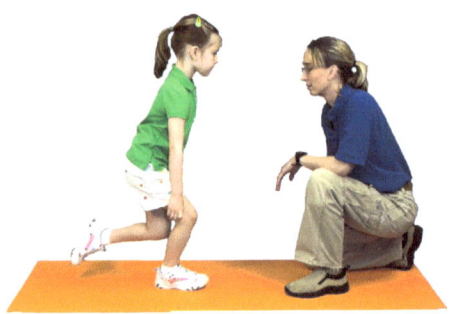

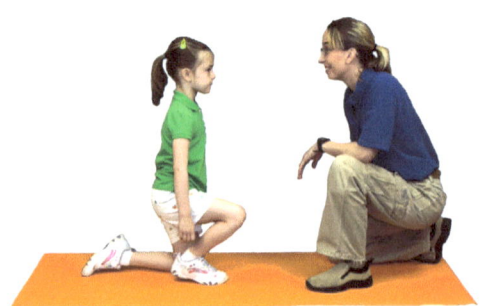

PEDIATRIC PHYSICAL THERAPY STRENGTHENING EXERCISES FOR THE KNEES

26. SQUATS WITH TRAINING BANDS

I love these bands. Using training bands with handles, I can perform squat to stands. I like trying this variation with the child leaning back more, farther from the hookup point and also more vertical, closer to the hookup point. Yes, a child can use her arms to assist, but that is what some kids need.

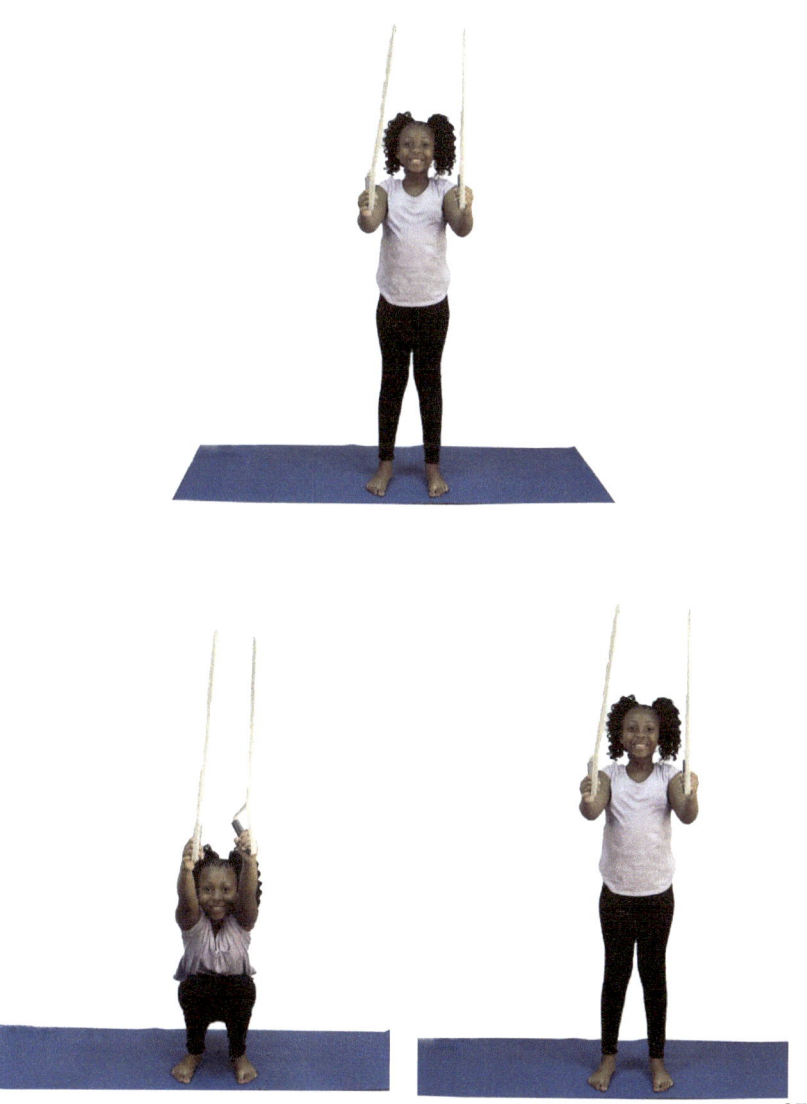

27. HALF KNEEL TO STAND WITH TRAINING BANDS

Another variation using the training bands to strengthen quads.

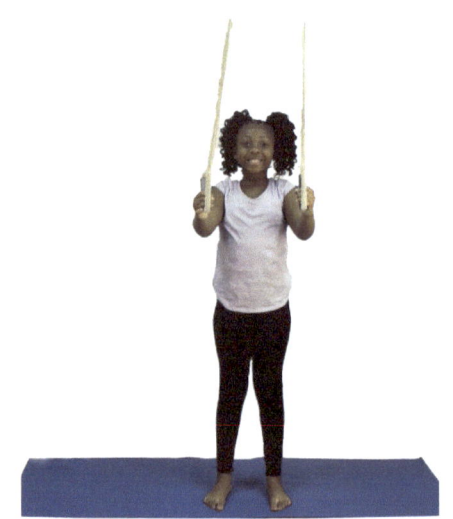

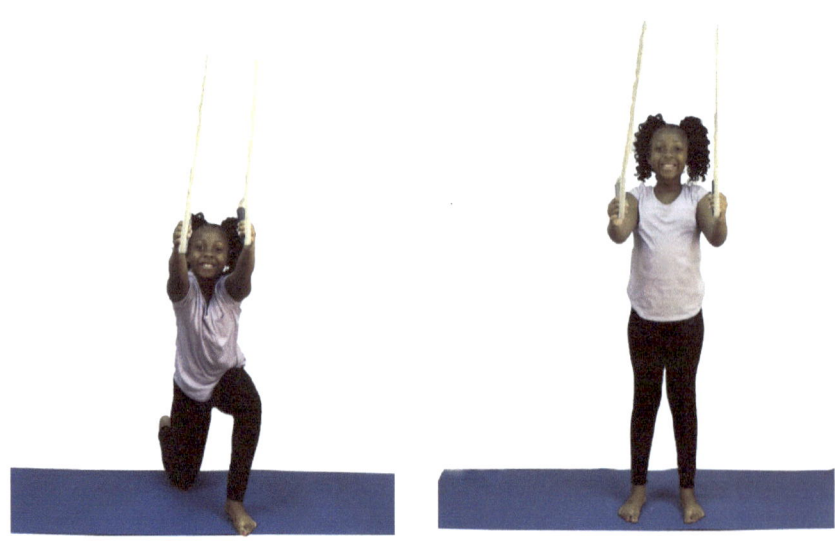

28. KICKING WITH HIP AND KNEE EXTENSION

With my clients with neurological issues, it is challenging for them to flex their hip keeping knee extension. These clients often have a steppage gait pattern. In this exercise, I am practicing keeping terminal knee extension as he swings forward his leg. If my client stands on a small bench, it is easier to clear the foot in the swing phase. For my clients with cerebral palsy, this movement is incredibly hard to motor plan and perform.

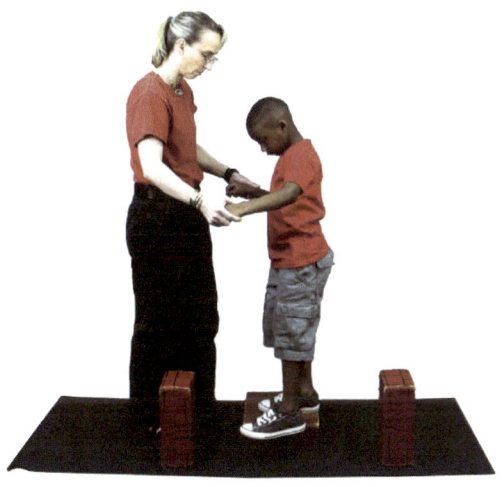

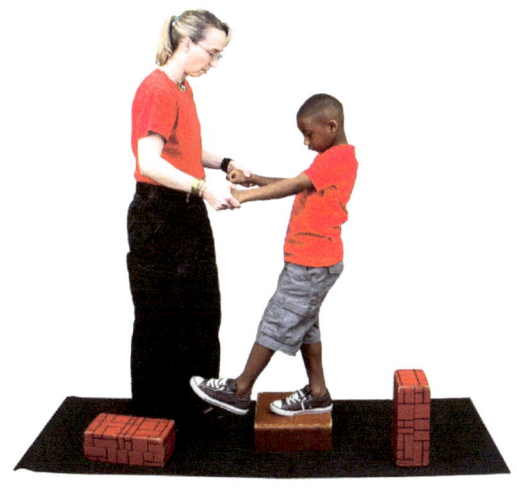

29. SLIDING/ROLLING A CAR FORWARD AND BACK

This is another activity targeting knee extension with active hip flexion/extension addressing gait abnormalities common with clients with a steppage gait pattern. Walking with this mass flexion/extension pattern is biomechanically inefficient, jarring to the joints, and loud, to say the least.

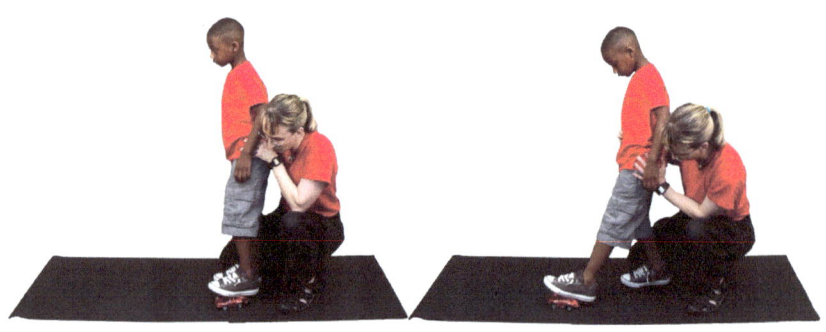

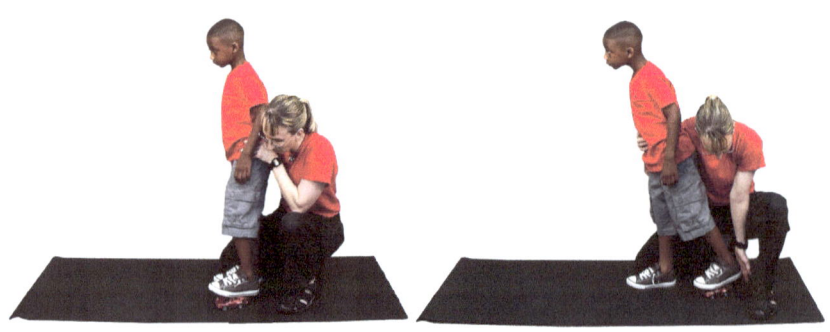

30. GLIDING ONE FOOT FORWARD AND BACK ON PAPER

If your client puts one foot on a paper, he can slide his foot forward and back. If he does not maintain the knee extension with the hip movement, then the paper does not slide with him. You don't need to have the stationary foot on the paper as pictured here.

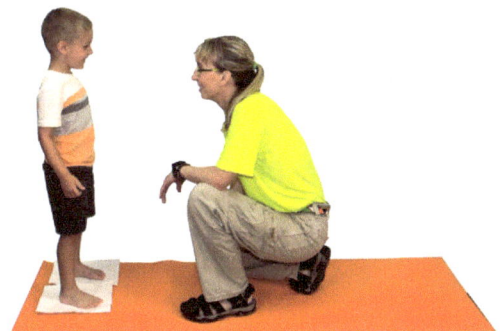

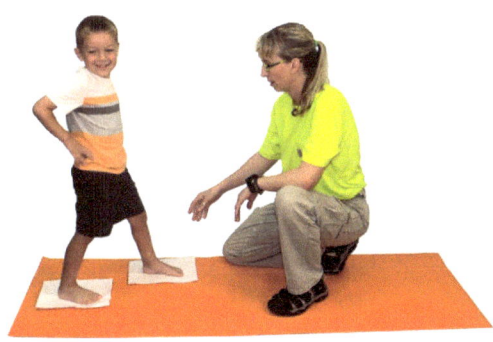

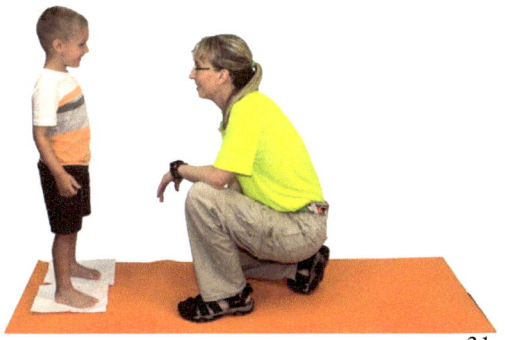

31. WALKING SLIDING PAPER UNDER FOOT

Yet another for knee extension with hip flexion. Perfect for the client with the steppage gait pattern to practice. This one is much harder than staying in one place.

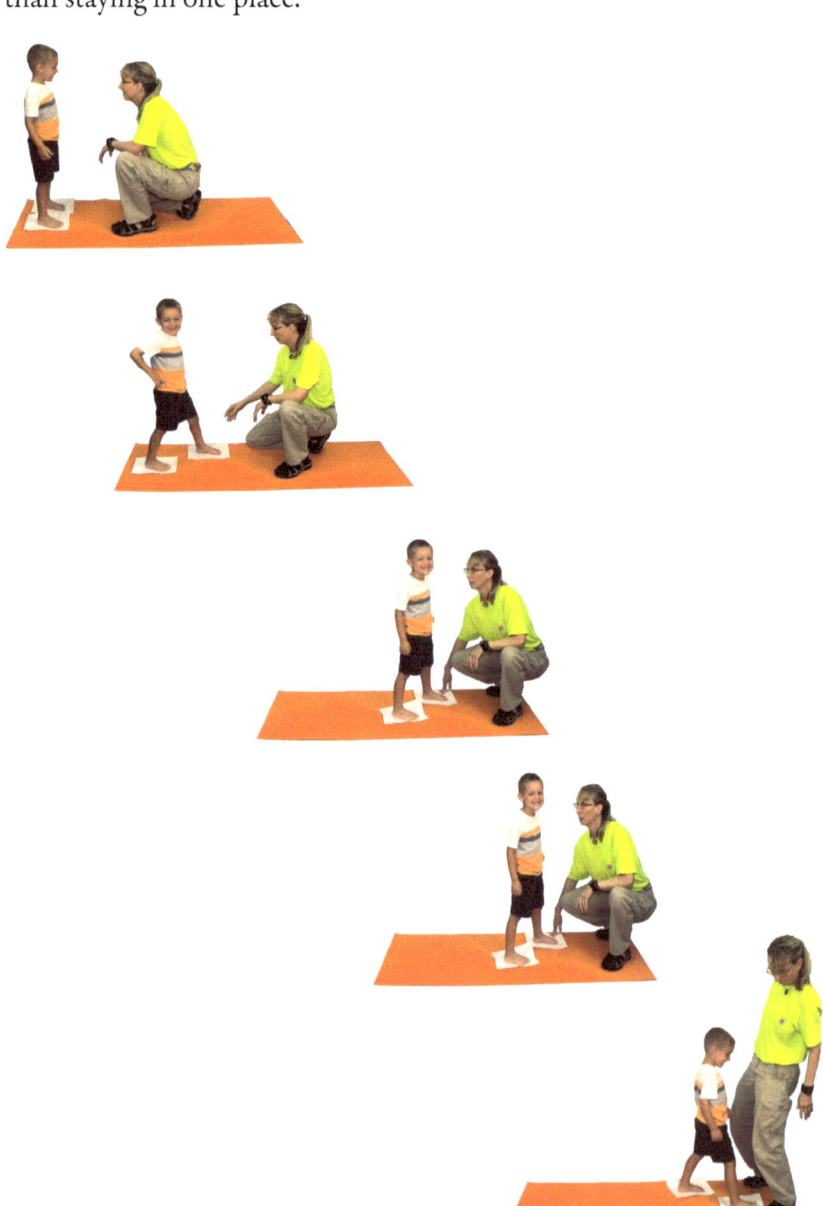

PEDIATRIC PHYSICAL THERAPY STRENGTHENING EXERCISES FOR THE KNEES

32. PUSH ME ON A STOOL OR A ROLLING DESK CHAIR

I am the one that loves this activity because I finally get to go for the ride! I sit on a rolling desk chair or stool. They can be hard for the child to simultaneously push and steer, but a challenge can be a good thing. Remember that pushing on hard floors like wood, or vinyl tile is much easier than carpet. If there is a sibling in the room, I usually let him or her take the ride. A parent is fun to push too. They often need to help by pulling some with his/her legs. Kids love when I return the favor and push them for an equal distance. I usually start off giving the child a ride, and then I take my turn.

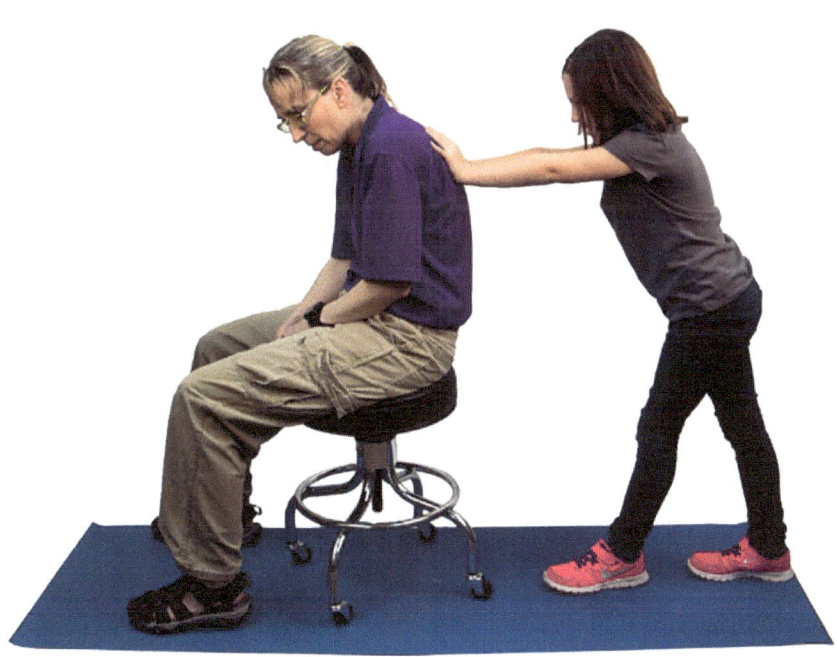

33. YOU PUSH ME ON THE SCOOTERBOARD

My comments from the previous activity still apply. I often will motivate the child by putting stacked blocks at the finish line. The person riding knocks down the blocks dramatically and with flare. All the crashing adds to the fun.

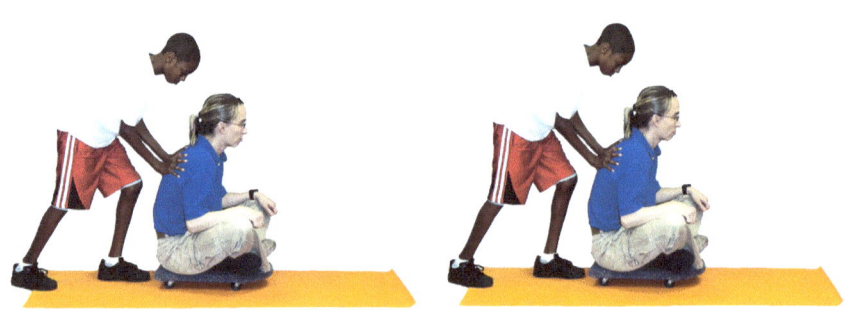

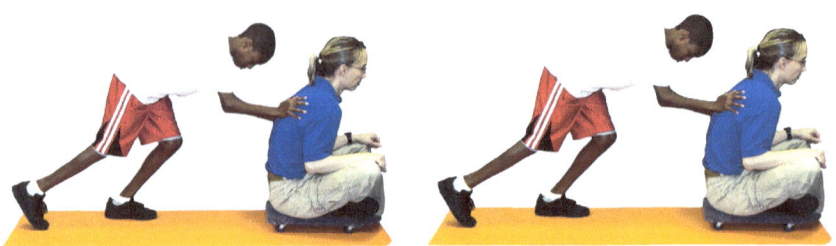

PEDIATRIC PHYSICAL THERAPY STRENGTHENING EXERCISES FOR THE KNEES

34. SCOOTERBOARD PUSH

I perform this activity frequently. The child stands behind the scooterboard and leans down and puts his hands on the scooterboard. He stays on his feet and pushes the scooterboard. I have the children go around a loop in our building. I usually grab another scooterboard and do the same with them. I have noticed that children often have trouble decelerating and stopping. Watch out! Your heels or the siblings' heels can get painfully ran over if you are not careful.

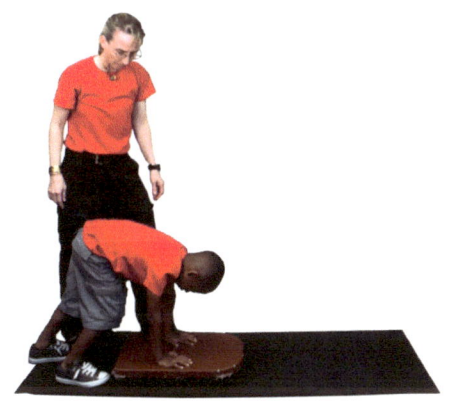

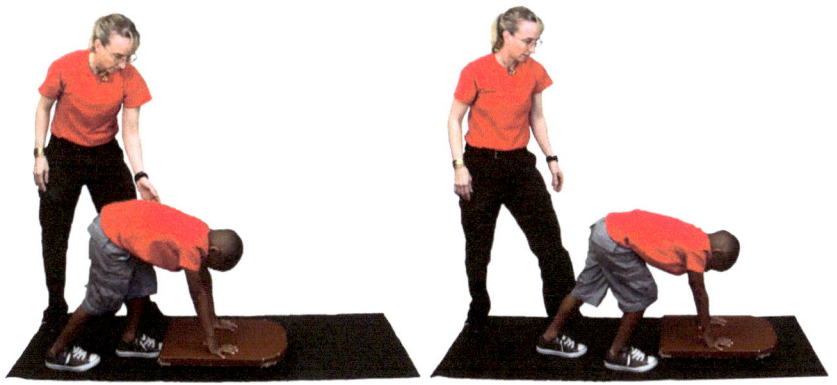

35. SCOOTERBOARD PUSH WITH BENCH

To make the previous activity a little easier, I often will put a 4" bench on top of the scooterboard. Assuming your scooterboard is rectangular like ours at the clinic, make sure the ends of the bench go to the front and back versus side to side. This arrangement makes it less likely for the bench to fall off the scooterboard. For less-skilled children, I may use a belt to cinch down the bench on the scooterboard.

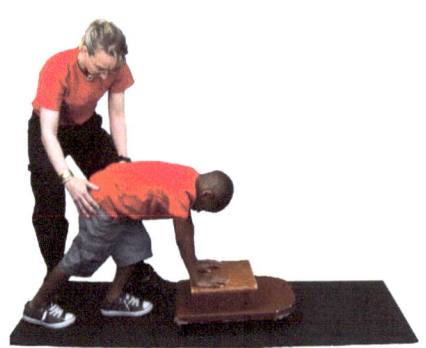

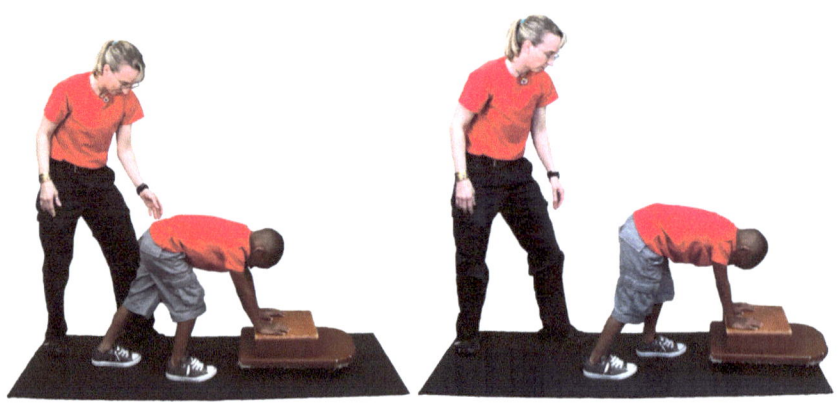

36. STEP UP AND DOWN

My clients are remarkably tolerant of this activity. Sometimes I use my benches like in this picture. However, most of the time, I have the child step up and down from folded mats. I know exactly how tall the mat is if I fold it once, twice, three or four times. By folding the mat, I can easily adjust the difficulty of this exercise. In my experience, with a child who is challenged by this activity, one inch can make a big difference. I will say that the Kaye Products adjustable benches (such as seen in this picture) are also easy to modify in height, so that would be my second choice. My clients with cerebral palsy who work on this activity usually have to be reminded to lean forward, so their head is over the knee stepping up. Others clients try to figure out how to pole vault over the front leg, getting little to no bend in the front leg.

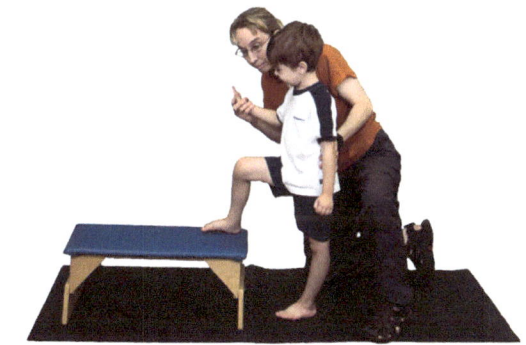

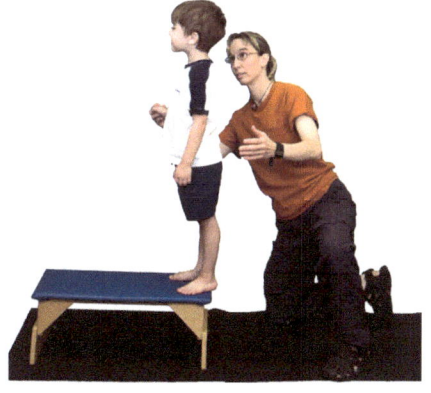

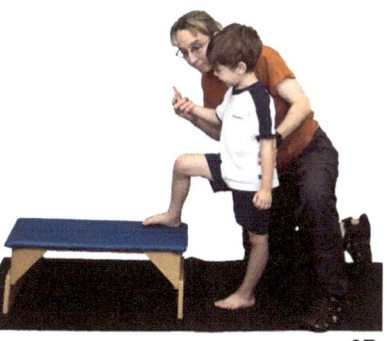

37. WALK UP STAIRS

To graduate the difficulty of this exercise, I progress from trunk support from behind, to two hands held support, to one hand on a rail and one hand held, to one hand held, to one hand on the rail, to one hand on a wall, to independently.

I have clients who can't walk or stand independently, but we practice the stairs. It is a terrific leg strengthening exercise. I support the child from behind and lift one leg (if she can't do it by herself) to the next step. I ask the child to push through the leading leg to ascend to the next step. Then I ask her to bring the trailing leg to the step the other foot is on. Then repeat. I usually do one flight of stairs leading with the left foot and then one flight of stairs leading with the right foot. I have to remind most of my clients with cerebral palsy to lean forward "nose over toes" instead of extending dangerously backward. With a client prone toward leaning back, I also remind the child to move her hand further up the rail after each step. "Step, Slide, Step, Slide." I like the child's hand to be one to two steps ahead of the step her feet are on.

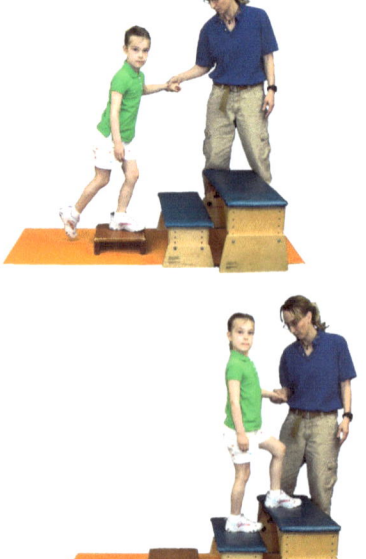
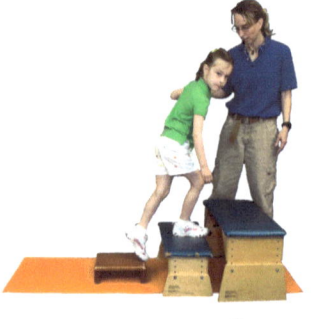
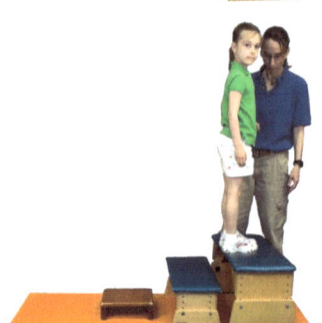

38. WALK DOWN STAIRS SLOWLY

I like to spot an ambulatory client who might fall on the stairs from behind. I keep my hands on the child's hips. I stay ready to pull the child back onto my lap if there is a problem. Only when I am pretty sure of a child's safety will I go in front to spot a child on stairs. For less skilled stair users, I always remind the client to hold onto the rail in front of her. They tend to let the arm holding the railing get behind them. They end up hanging off the rail instead of propping forward on it as they go down the stairs. I emphasize going down the stairs slowly to encourage eccentric contractions of the quadriceps muscle.

With clients who can't walk or stand independently, I still practice stairs. I support the child from behind, weight shift her to take a step, and then I help to lower her to the next step. She brings the trailing leg to the step that the other foot is on, and repeat. I usually do one flight of stairs leading with the left foot and the next with right. Going down is easier than up. Being able to descend stairs with assistance is an important skill. If the elevator isn't working, at least you can get the child down the stairs. I've had to do that more than a few times. So much better to walk, than carry, a heavy child down the stairs.

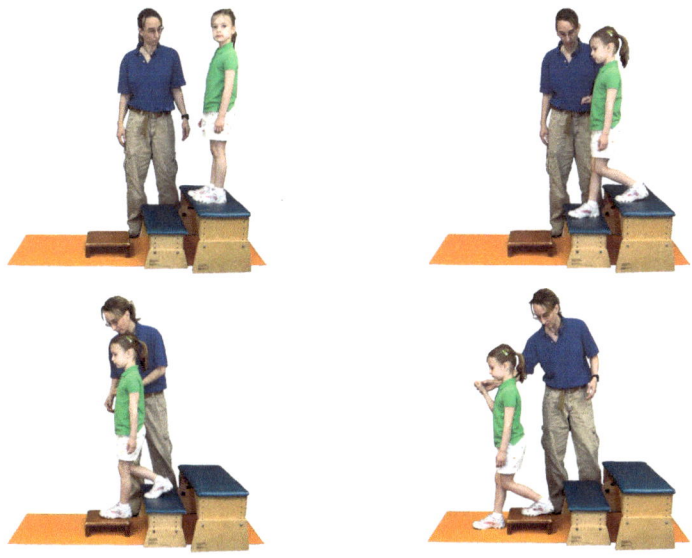

39. BACKWARD STEP UP AND DOWN

I perform this exercise sometimes with a single bench in my room, working for repetitions to get concentric and eccentric quads. I progress from trunk support from the front, to two hands held support, to one hand on a wall grip and one hand held, to one hand held, to one hand on a wall, to independently to graduate the difficulty of this exercise. When using the bench, sometimes I have the child do the entire movement starting with standing backward to the bench, stepping back putting one foot and then the second on the bench. Sometimes I let the child leave one foot on the bench behind him, so all he has to do is move the other leg up and down.

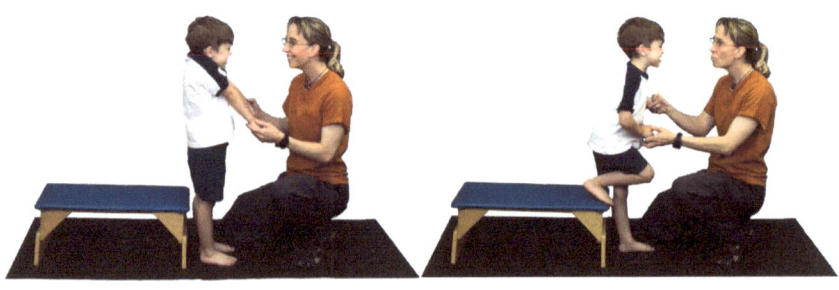

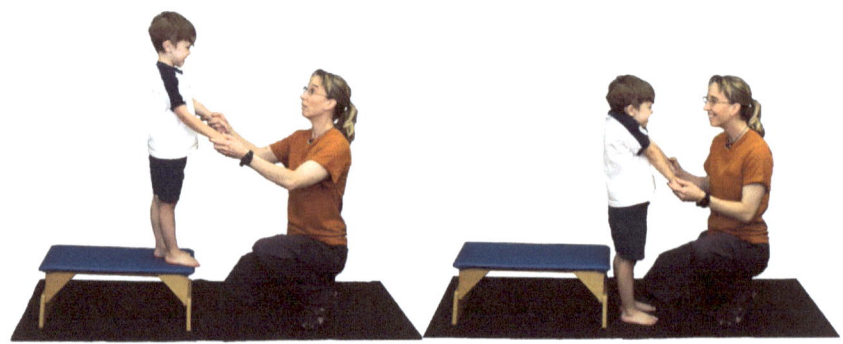

40. BACKWARD UP AND DOWN THE STAIRS

I like the stairs, better than the bench. Since I have 20 steps at my facility between floors, that guarantees me 20 reps. Encouraging a child to do 20 repetitions on a bench is trickier. Backward down the stairs emphasizes eccentrics, and upstairs works concentric quads. I progress the difficulty similar to the previous exercise. Most kids don't give me a hard time with backward up or down the stairs.

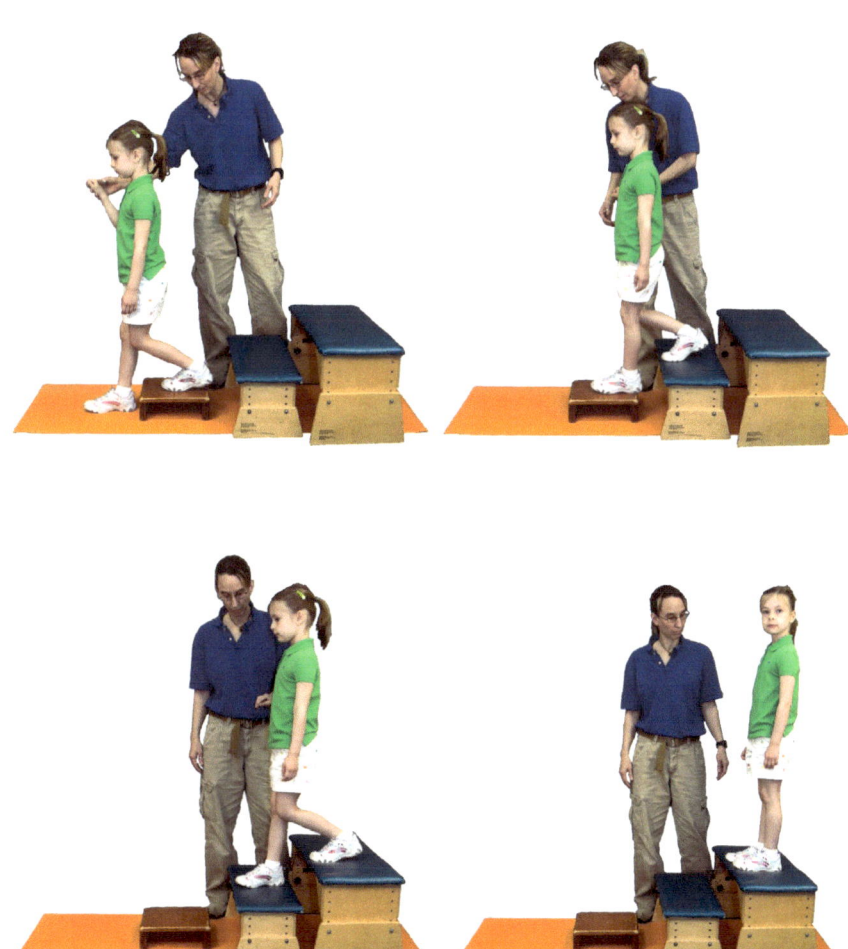

41. HURDLE JUMP

I start low and work my way taller. The taller or the wider the hurdle is, the harder the obstacle is to traverse. I often start with a 1" thick pole, progressing to a 2" x 4" board flat to get a 2" tall obstacle. Then I put the board on end to make it 4" tall. If I go higher, I usually have the child jump over a rope. I hold one end of the rope and drape the other end over a bench on the other side. Setting it up this way allows no injury if the child misses. I emphasize a two-foot take-off and landing. Kids with a stronger leg, lift first the weaker leg and then jump off the more capable leg for more of a "leap" than a jump.

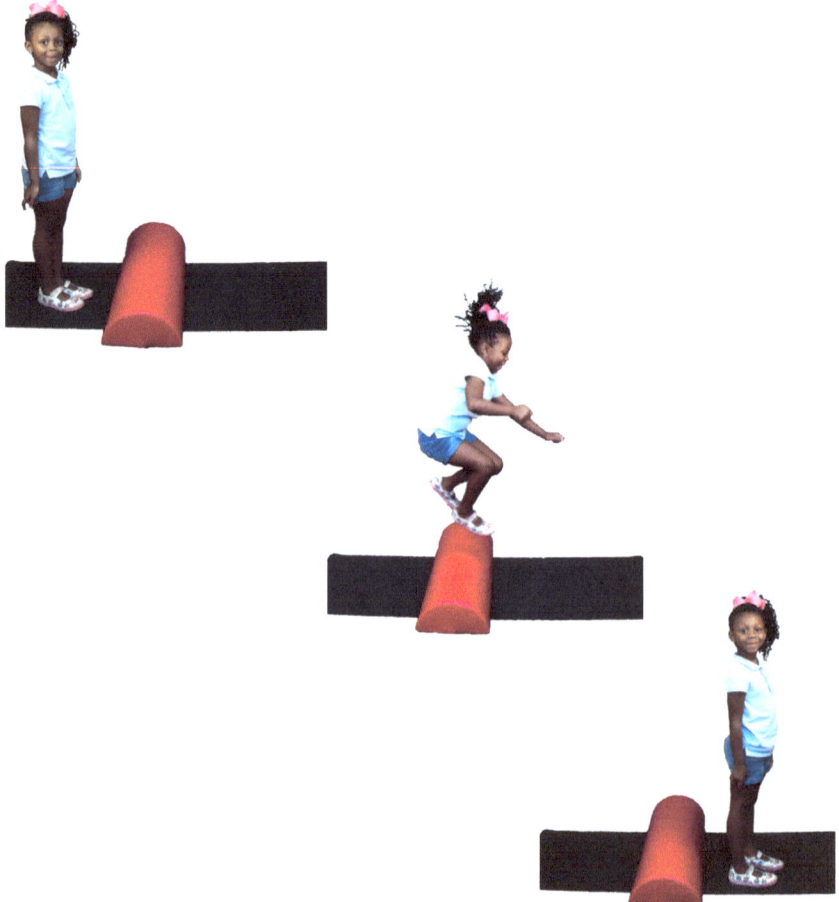

42. JUMP ONTO

Another variation on this activity is to have the child jump up onto a surface. Obviously, the higher the surface, the harder this activity is. I use my folding mats for this trick 99% of the time. I start with the lowest one-ply mat and work my way up. Once I have found the correct height, I ask for ten repetitions.

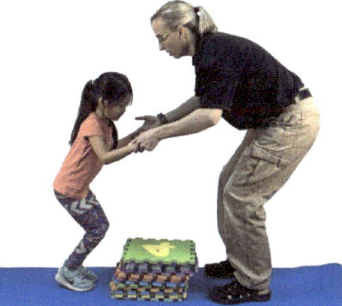

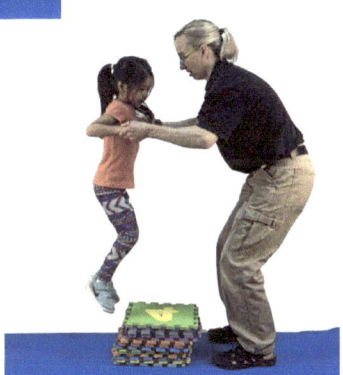

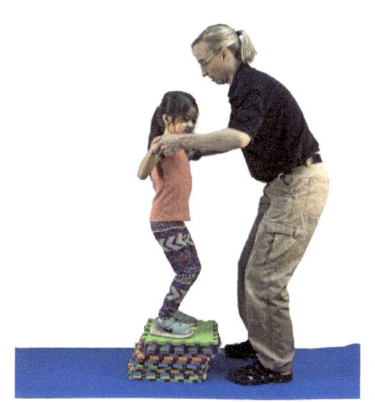

43. LUNGES WITH 1-2 HANDS HELD

Here my model needed support to get back up to standing again from the lunge position. I usually mark on my carpet with Velcro lines where I want my client to start, to step out to, and to step back to in one big step. I start with small distances and work further. I try to get the child to put the knee down to the floor of the non-stepping leg.

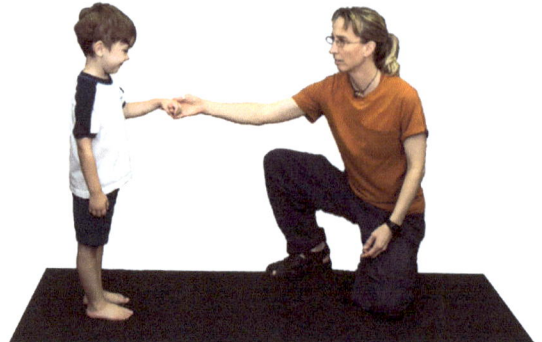

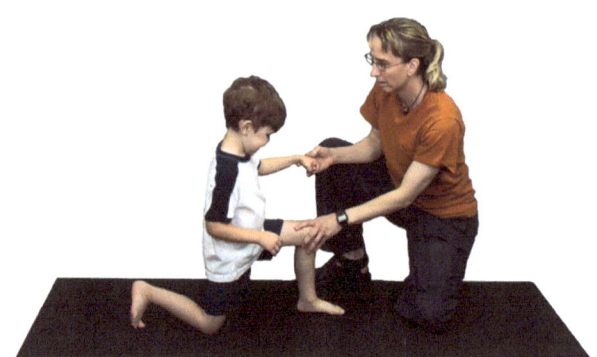

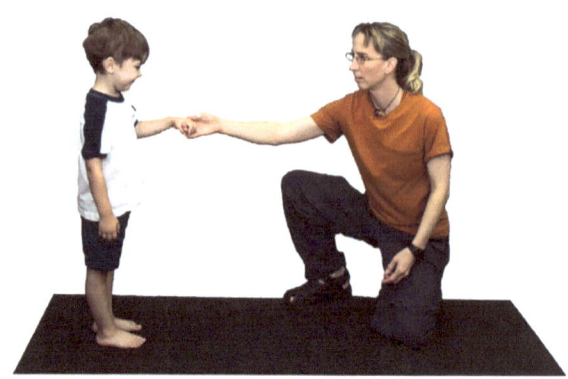

44. LUNGES WITH NO SUPPORT

This is the independent version of the previous exercise. Here I am using carpet squares to indicate where I want her to step to and back to. These are very hard. Start with smaller step lengths and work toward longer.

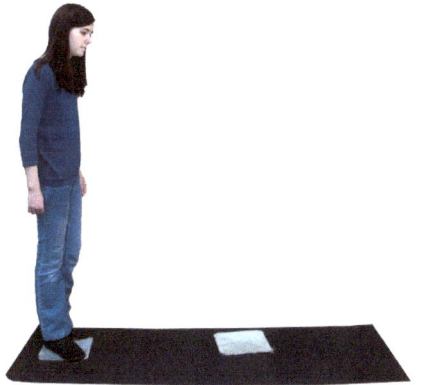

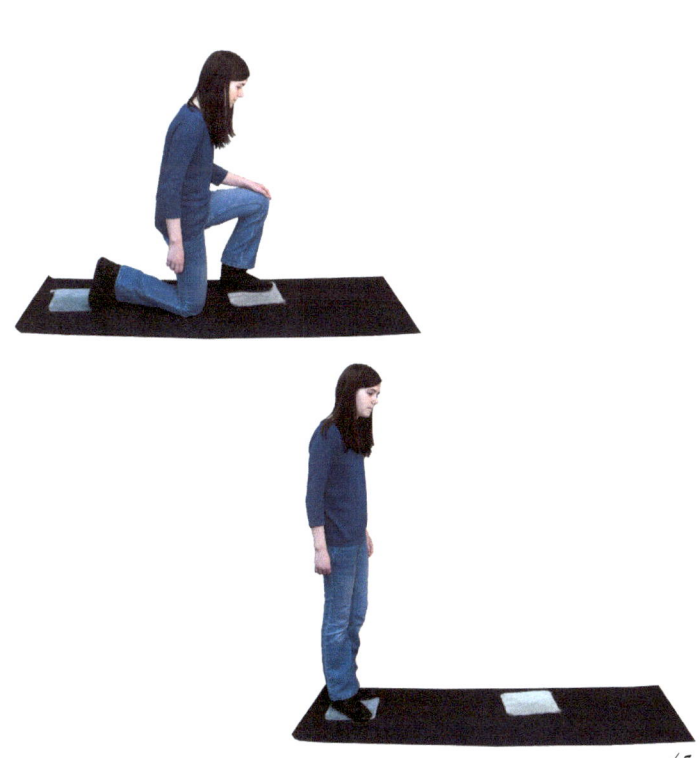

45. WALL SITS

I know, I know, collective groan from all the children I have ever made do this exercise. It is a tough one, and there had better be something really fun afterward. Sometimes I go for repetitions up and down. In other cases, I ask the child to go down and hold the wall sit for one to ten seconds. Miserable perhaps, but a great strengthening exercise. I do the exercise along with the child if I think he won't fall down without my assistance. If I think the child might collapse, I sit on the floor in front of the child facing him. I put up my index fingers and ask the child to dip down until he touches his knees to my finger tips. This seems to work best as it gives the child a target. It also puts me in position to catch the child by blocking his descent at his knees. I have a child with a myopathy who can only control the first ten degrees of a wall sit. He collapses if he tries to slide lower. So we work the range he can safely control. Since he is bigger, I put a 10 inch bench waiting under him between his feet and the wall to catch him if he falls.

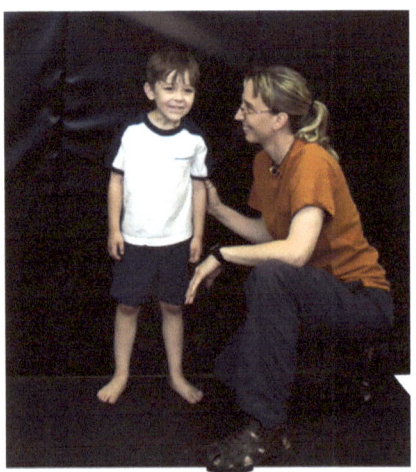 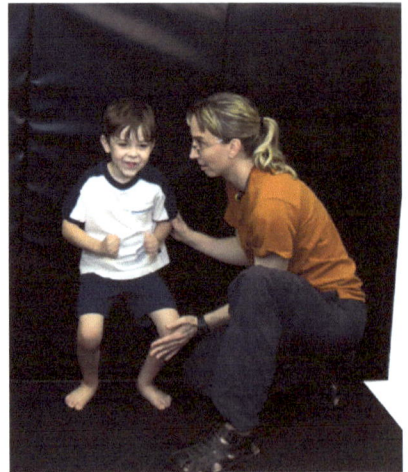

46. WALL TALLS

For the crouch walkers, I do almost the reverse of a classic wall sit. I let the child stand with her back to the wall with her typical knee/hip flexion. I sit on the floor in front of her facing the child. I put my palms on her knees, and I say, "Stand up taller, straightening your hips and knees to get your knees off of my fingers." As the child extends her hips/knees, I reposition my hands to touching her knees again and repeat. At the child's end range, I may have the child keep her knees off my hands and time how long she is successful.

I use another variation of this exercise with children with quadriplegic cerebral palsy who have difficulty getting end range knee/hip extension in standing. I stand the child with her back on the wall. I hold her hands and lift the child to a less crouched position pushing with my knees through her knees until we find the tallest she can stand with assistance. With convenient pre-placed Velcro strips on the wall, I have a helper Velcro a box to the wall touching the top of the child's head. Then I unblock the child's knees while still holding the hands. The child immediately sinks. Her head is no longer touching the Velcro'd box. I ask the child to push with her legs so that she is tall enough again to touch her head to the box, either momentarily for a certain number of repetitions or a specified duration.

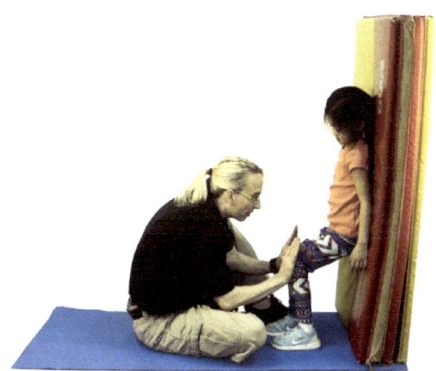
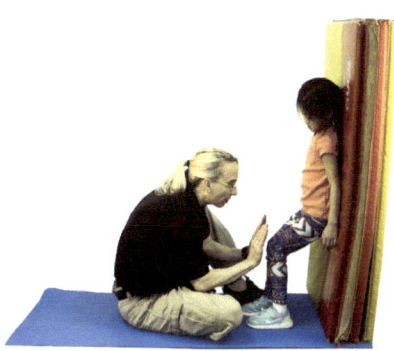

47. KNEE KNOCK DOWNS

This exercise works both eccentric/concentric plantarflexors and quadriceps. A taller block is easier to knock down than a shorter one. I usually start with the target touching the child's toes and then move the block further forward as the child is successful for a more significant challenge. This activity is hard on two legs and twice as hard on one leg. No hands held is much harder.

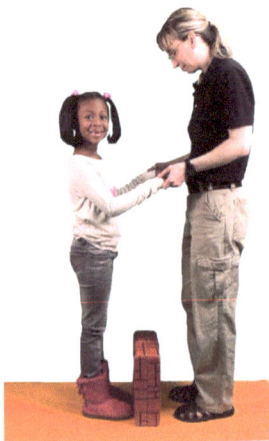

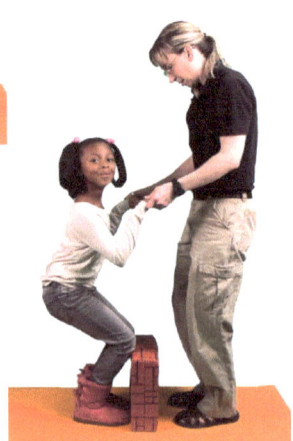

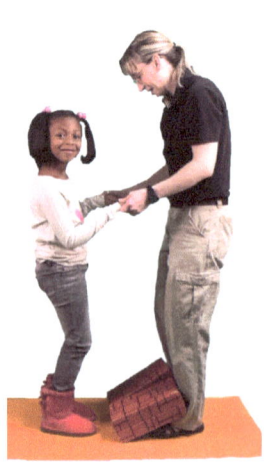

48. ONE POLE, ONE LEG, PICK UP

Kids like or at least tolerate this game. No poles? Then a doorknob or the corner of a table works as well. For more challenge, I don't stabilize the pole at all and let the client work through the instability. For the most advanced clients, I still use the pole, but I don't let my client hold onto it. I have children pick up either the swimming pool rings that children dive for or bracelets. Kids like the bracelets because if the child spins the ring as it is released, it will helicopter spin, in a most satisfying manner, down the pole. If a child is having a hard time, I help by supporting the leg that the child has lifted. If the client needs a little more stability, then I have the child lift the leg closest to the pole for a broader base of support. For a little more challenge, I have the child lift the foot furthest from the pole. I have found that if I put the ring forward a little further, I get a little more knee flexion than if the ring is close to the child's foot.

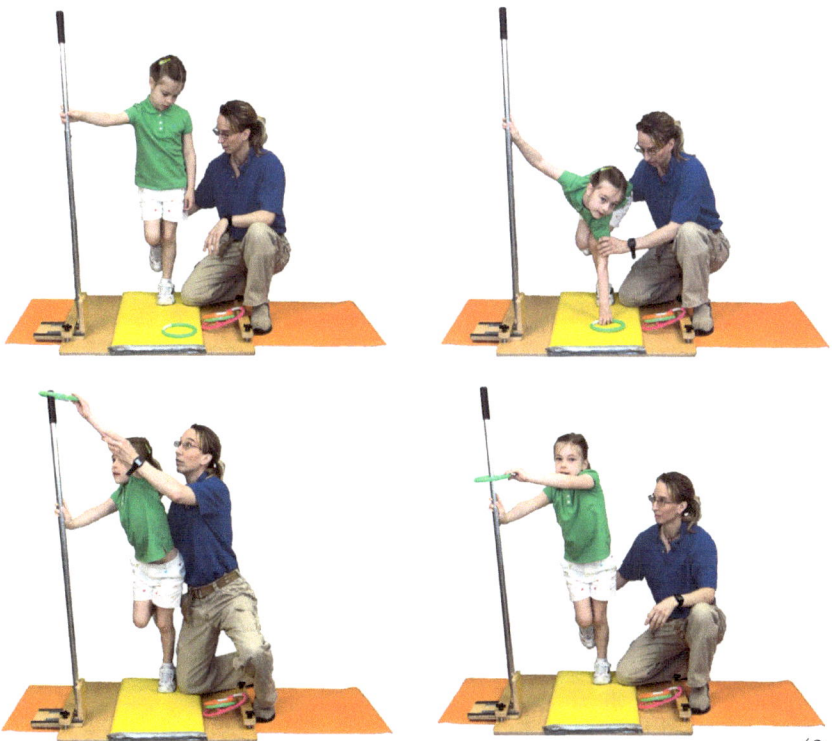

49. SIDE PICK UP, ONE FOOT ON A BENCH

This exercise is particularly useful for clients with hemiplegia. By putting one foot up on a bench, the client is immediately more likely to put more weight on the foot on the floor. That said, I have seen more than a few kids try to figure out how to perform this exercise without putting more weight on the foot on the floor. In this case, I support the knee on the down leg to guide the weight shift to the side for picking up the object. More weight is shifted to the down leg as the other foot is put on a progressively higher bench. Some clients need trunk support, a hand held, or a bench in front of them to stabilize to complete this activity. This is where toys with pieces are wonderful.

Often I stand the child at a taller bench with something like a ten-piece puzzle on it. I put puzzle pieces down on the floor for the child to pick up. He leans down, grabs the piece, and stands up to put the piece in the puzzle on the bench in front of the child. I may initially not put the toy as low as the ground. I may not even put one foot up relative to the other. I measure progress by how close to the floor I can hold/place the toy and the child still manage to pick it up and return to upright. Any child who can cruise is ready to start working on this game, albeit with a bench/furniture in front of him. If the child is stronger and has more balance, then I perform this exercise without the bench in front like in this picture.

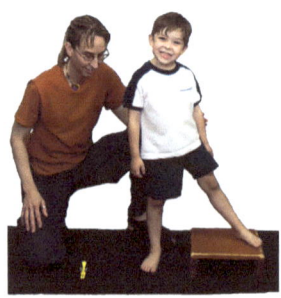 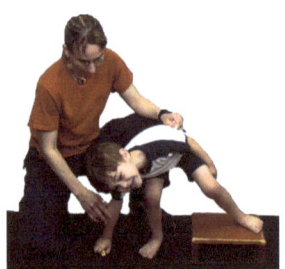 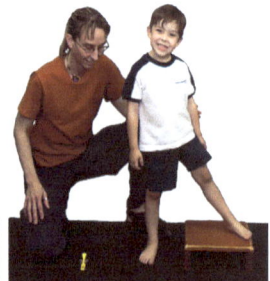

50. PICK UP IN FRONT WITH FOOT UP IN BACK

This activity is challenging and doesn't win me any points with the kids. A taller bench in the back makes this harder. I usually don't place the back foot up any higher than the kid's knee. I often have to remind the child that I only want the toe of the foot in back on the bench-not the whole foot flat. I love this activity because it works on balance, as well as hip and knee extensors and plantarflexors. You get eccentric muscle contractions on the way down and concentric on the way up. Toys with pieces are the key. Here the child is picking up an oreo cookie-shaped puzzle piece. I see more flexion at the three joints when the toy is placed further out relative to the child's foot.

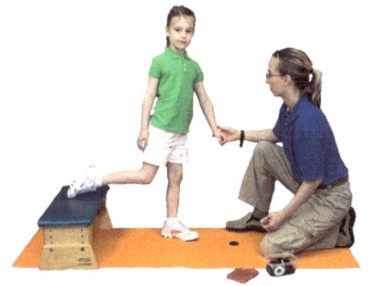

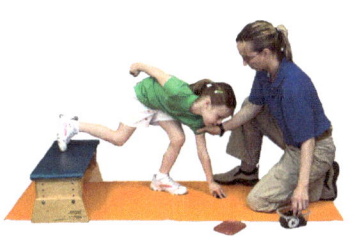

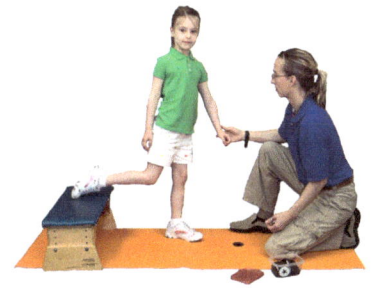

51. PICK UP IN FRONT WITH FOOT ON SLANT IN BACK

This activity is similar to the exercise in which the child picks up a toy with one foot back on the bench. This can be easier or harder depending on how steep you make the slant. I typically use a mat leaning against a wall. This activity is easier with a lower incline and harder with a steeper incline. It usually takes me a few reps to determine the correct slant, and then I try to get ten repetitions.

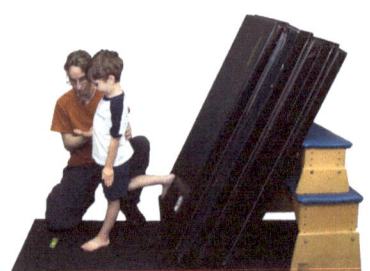

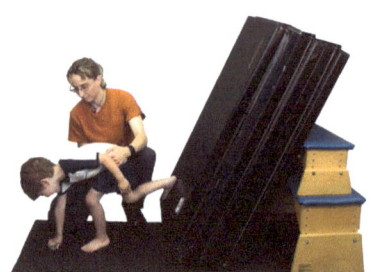

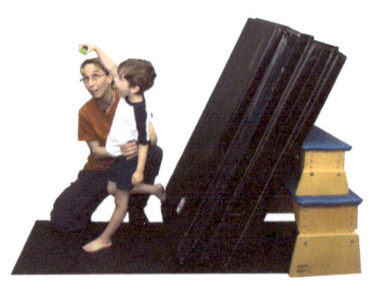

PEDIATRIC PHYSICAL THERAPY STRENGTHENING EXERCISES FOR THE KNEES

52. ONE LEG PICK UP BELOW

This exercise shows the progression of the one leg pick Encourage more knee movement by having the client pick up an object lower than her foot. Only a few of my higher-level clients with hemiplegia can perform this activity hands-free, but the majority can't get to this level without additional assistance.

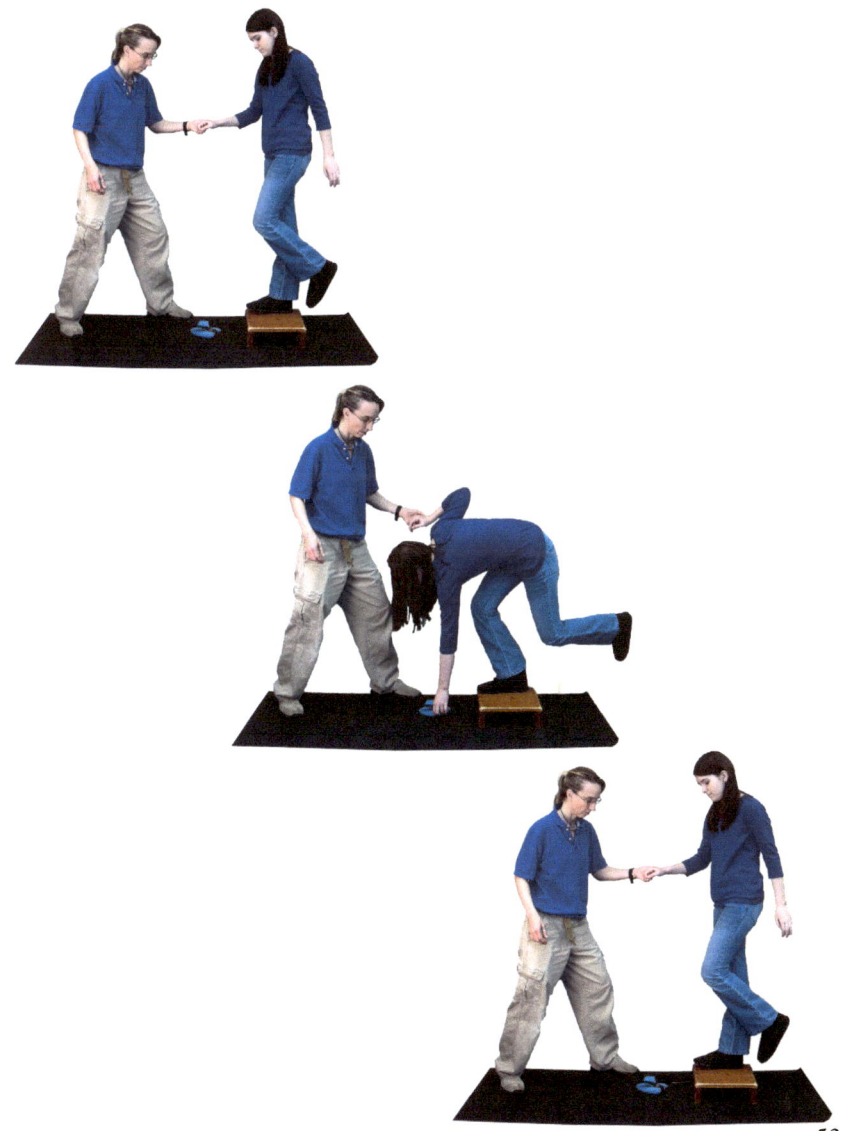

53. DIP KICKS WITH TWO POLE SUPPORT

I love this exercise, and I am always continuously amazed that kids don't hate it. I love the poles with this exercise. I have also used one railing and a hand held, but upright poles are perfect because a child of any height can grab the pole at the right height for them. I start with two poles and then work to one pole.

A taller bench makes this harder as well. Technically, the differential in height between the bench and toy she is kicking determines the difficulty level. To make this activity harder, I lower the toy relative to the bench the child is standing on. If that is not enough, then I make the bench higher.

I should note that the first thing a child tries is simply to plantarflex the kicking foot to knock over the toy. You'll have to put the toy low enough that the child has to bend her hip/knee. Also, note that if a child has an ankle-foot orthosis with a plantarflexion stop, then you won't need to make the toy as low. The child can't plantarflex her foot to reach the toy. The range will come only from hip and knee movement.

It never hurts to have a spot on this activity. I usually am down low, placing the toy to be kicked, so I am not in an advantageous position to spot the child in case there is a loss of balance. So I will often have a parent stand nearby to guard as well.

PEDIATRIC PHYSICAL THERAPY STRENGTHENING EXERCISES FOR THE KNEES

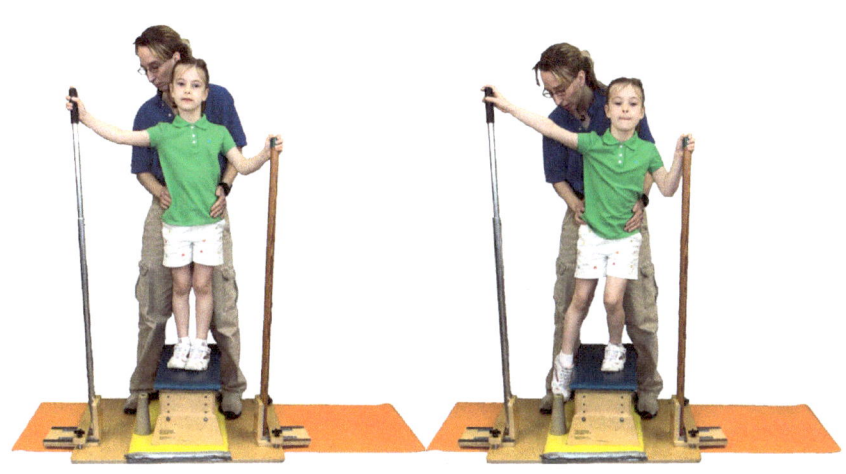

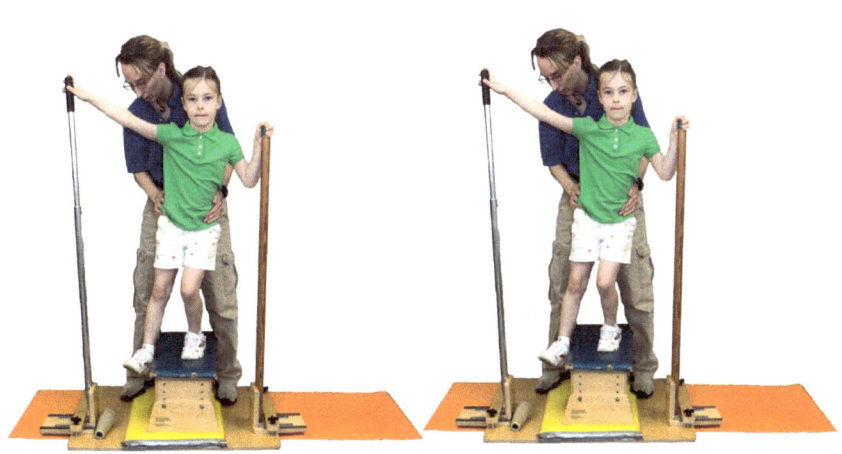

54. DIP KICKS WITH ONE POLE SUPPORT

I perform this exercise with the following in decreasing order of support: with one hand holding one pole, with one hand held, with one hand on the wall with my client facing sideways standing on top on the bench. If one hand is supported, I strategically put the pole on the side of the stance leg if I think the child needs a narrower base of support. I put the pole on the kicking leg side for a broader base of support. If I need to make this activity even harder, I may put the bench close to the wall but ask the child only to use it in an emergency.

I also modify the difficulty of this activity by changing the distance the client has to dip to kick the object. I can make the bench higher or the block lower. The client should kick and knock down the object but not touch the floor. I like foam blocks/animals or stacked cones/cups because I can make the distance that she has to dip down harder by merely removing one cone/cup from the stack. I could also have put my client on a taller bench. However, it is not uncommon that my clients lose their balance on this activity. If I don't have a second person to spot for safety, then I would use lower objects to increase the dip distance instead of using a taller bench.

If I find the perfect support level, then I can modify the difficulty by having her dip down repeatedly touching the hippo 2,3,4,5, up to 10 times before returning to the resting position on the bench with the kicking leg. In this case, I have to hold the hippo in place to keep it from being kicked away. Be wary of the potential hand smash!

Even on clients with one side that is clearly better at this activity, such as a client with hemiplegia, I will often let the client perform a few repetitions on their less/uninvolved side first. This allows them to get the feel of the movement before trying it with their more challenging side. I document how low the client can go with the less and the more involved side.

PEDIATRIC PHYSICAL THERAPY STRENGTHENING EXERCISES FOR THE KNEES

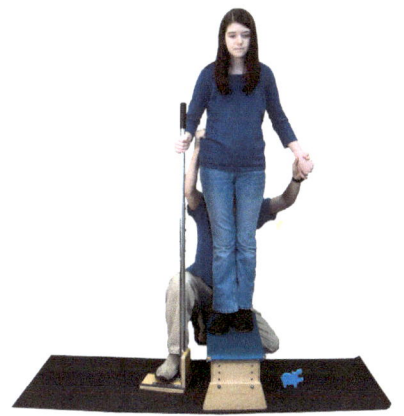

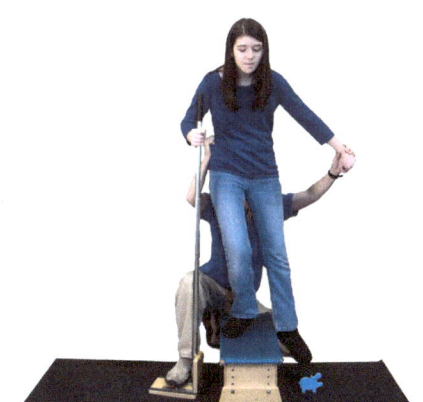

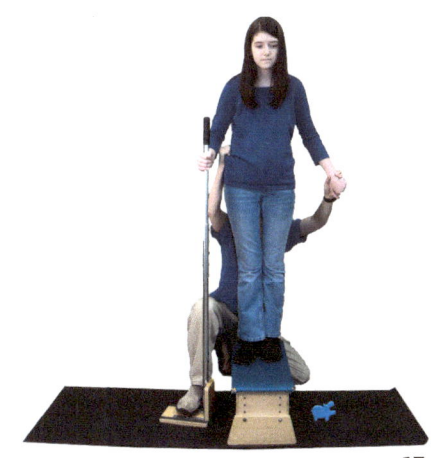

55. HOP ONE FOOT ON BENCH

On this exercise, hip extensors, plantarflexors, and knee extensors are working. If you want this to be a knee extension exercise, ask your child to make a preparatory knee bend on the leg on the floor before hopping to encourage knee extension. I can imagine my hand right at the knee and giving the verbal cue to "Bend and Hop!" Many of my children with significant weakness on one side, such as clients with hemiplegia, cheat something horrible on this exercise. I conceived of this activity to try to get work on the leg standing on the floor. But if that leg is quite weak, it is not uncommon for a child to weight shift to the leg on the bench and get the lift-off from that leg. In which case, I hold hands with the child and facilitate the weight shift to the leg on the floor. I will also note that the child hopping for this photo series is significantly exaggerating the hop so we can catch it on camera. I am usually satisfied with the foot simply clearing the floor.

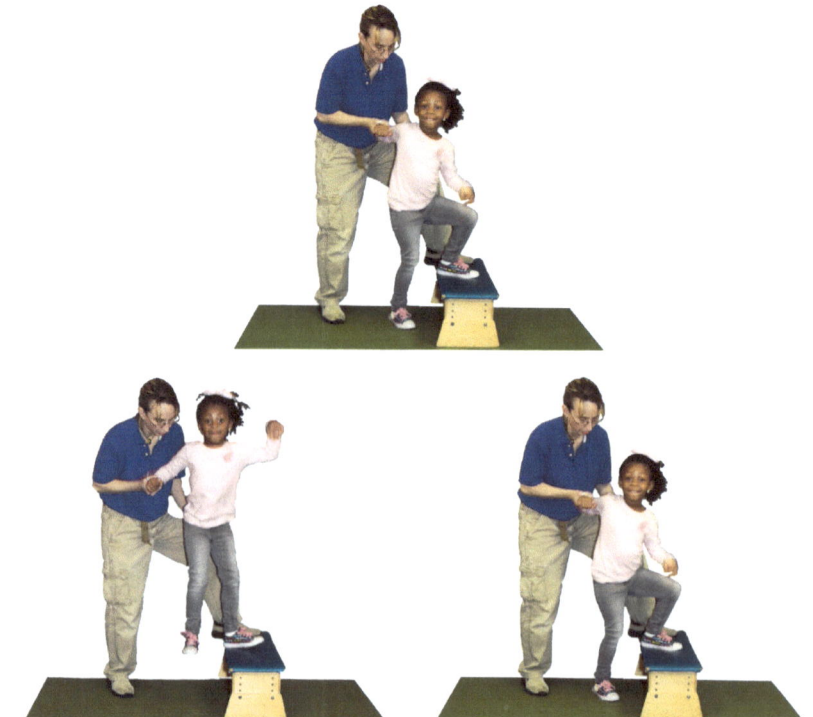

56. LAME DOGS

I can usually get children to do this one time, and then they remember how hard it was after that. In this exercise, your client hops along on her hands and one back leg like a dog who has a hurt back leg. Since legs are longer than arms, the child has to bend the weight-bearing leg, which sets her up for quadriceps and hip extensors to help out. This movement is difficult. For encouragement, I always do the exercise along with my clients. We have a long hall at work, so we lame dog down the hall, take a rest, and lame dog back.

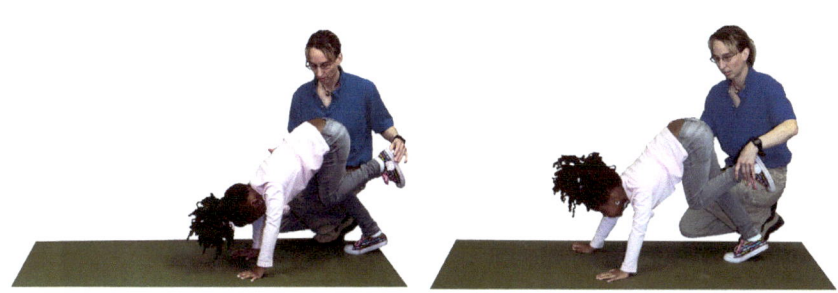

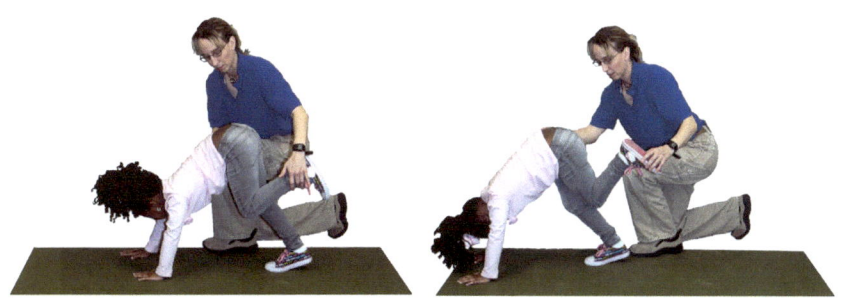

57. SKIP STEPS UP STAIRS

My kids are usually so proud to get to this exercise. They think it is cool. I either let a child hold two rails, one rail or let them try it independently. I strongly prefer to do this exercise on a real set of stairs. We have 20 steps between floors at work so I can get 10 reps by going just one flight.

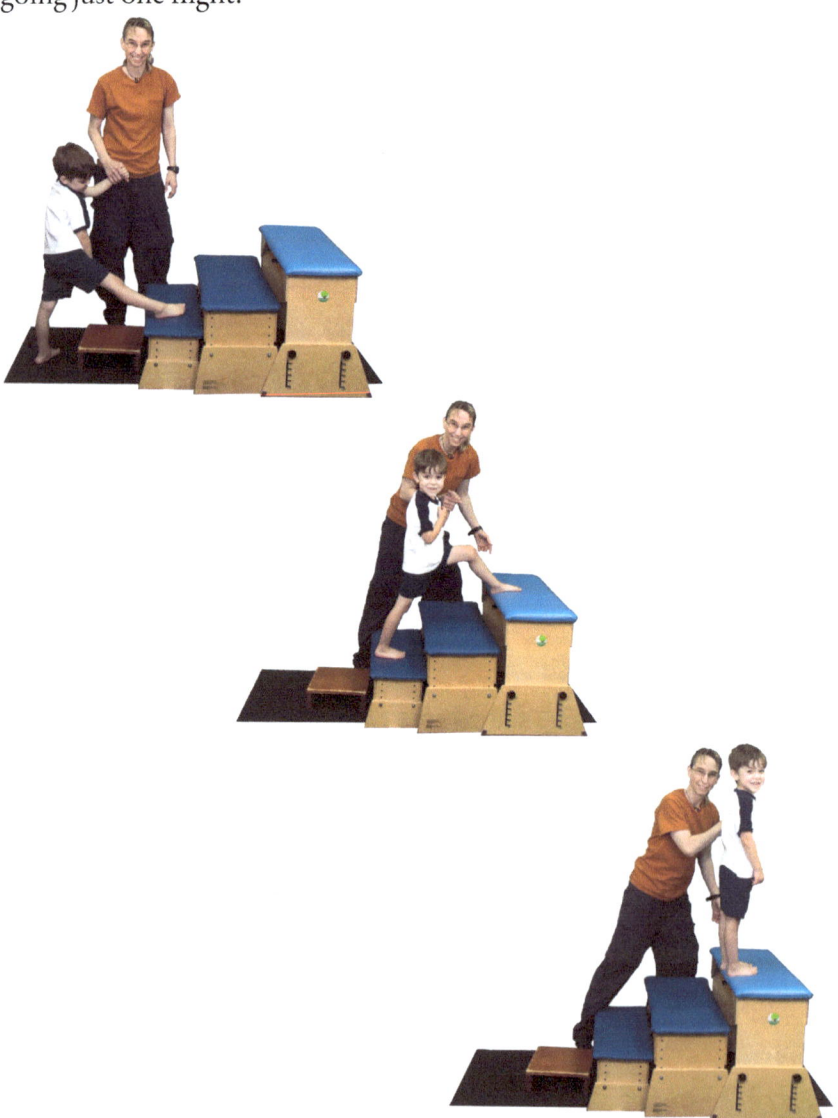

58. JUMP UP STAIRS

This exercise falls into the category of activities that the kids think are cool only the first time they try it. However, jumping up the stairs is hard. I try not to do this exercise if I don't think the child is ready. It is really easy to not jump high enough and clobber your shin on the next step. Never popular. I start with two hands on the rail (one on each side), then one hand, then some kids are good enough to try this with no hands on the railing. Since this height is extreme, kids usually recruit help at the ankle, knee, and hip. It is a great lower body work out.

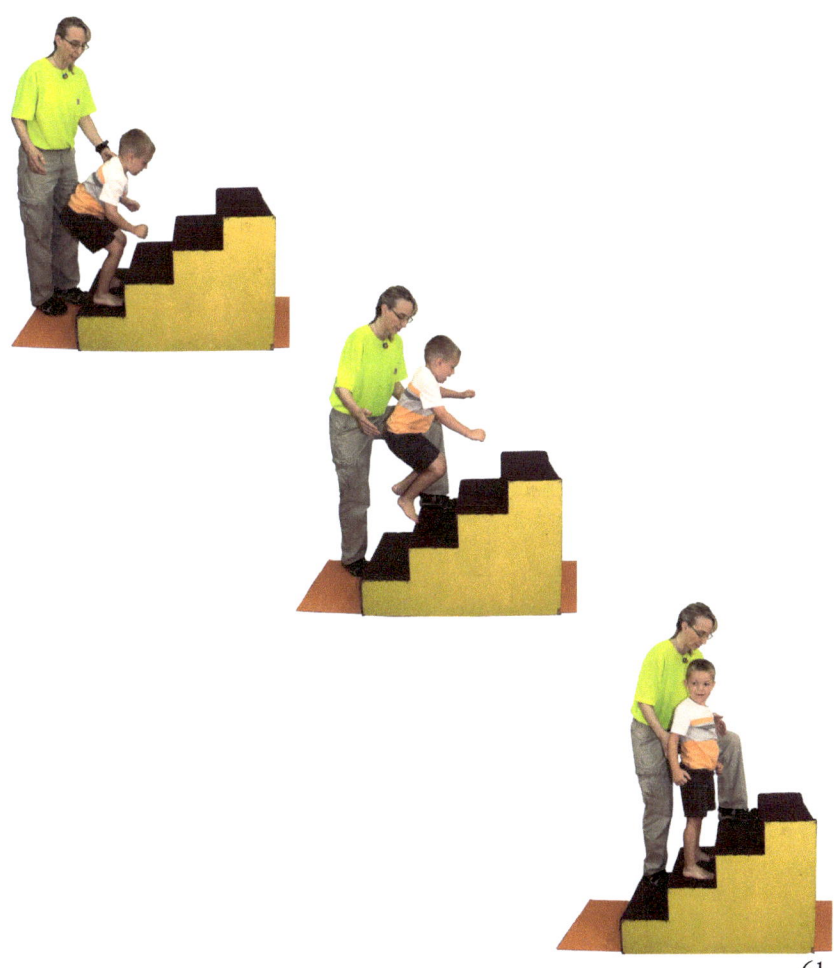

59. HOP UP STEPS

Similar to the previous exercise, but on one foot. If the child has a stronger leg, I always let her get the feel of this movement first with the better leg. The chance of hitting the shin is much higher now, so fade the support cautiously.

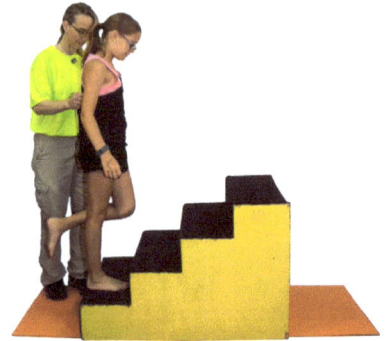

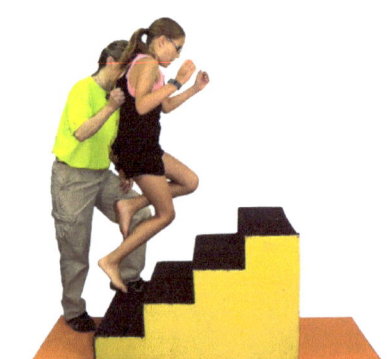

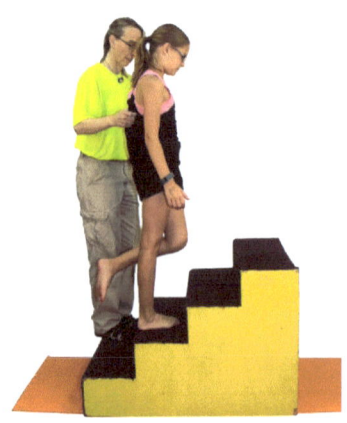

60. TALL KNEEL LEAN BACKS

Start with arms free and work toward arms crossed on chest. I usually put my hand behind the child as a target. I can also catch the child if she goes too far. This movement produces a forceful quad contraction. I stabilize the legs to assist.

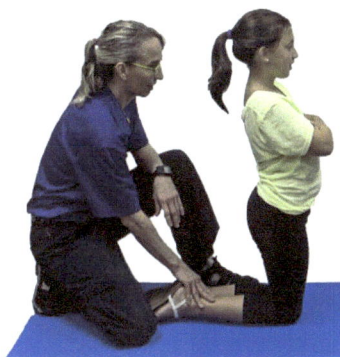

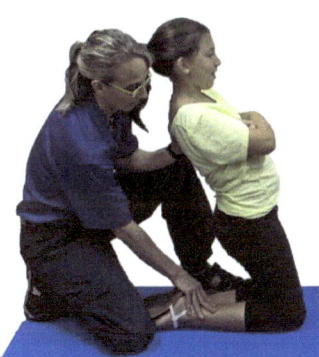

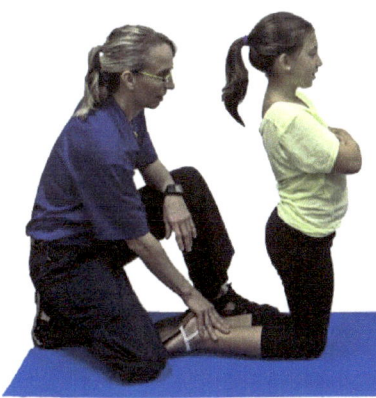

61. TALL KNEEL LEAN BACKS, ARMS UP

Putting the arms overhead just made the lever arm longer, making a tough exercise even tougher!

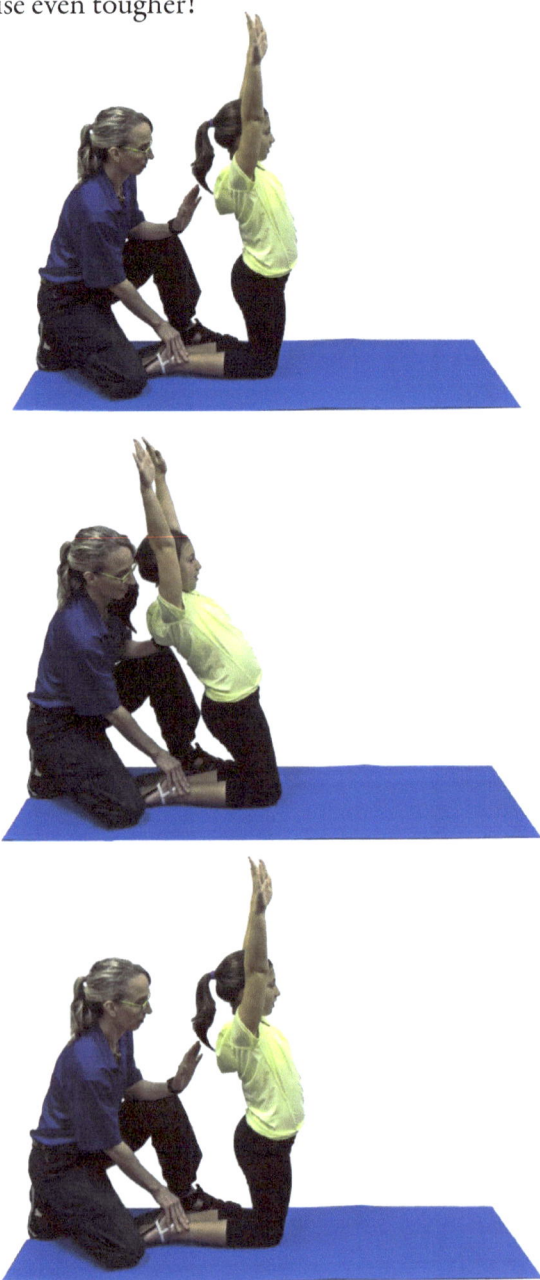

62 LUNGE WALKS

Instead of having children lunge forward and back ten times on one side and then ten times on the other, you could have the child do lunge walks instead. If I am asking my client to do this exercise, I always struggle through and perform it as well.

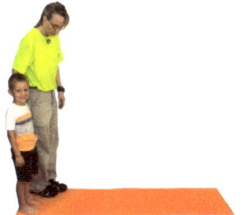

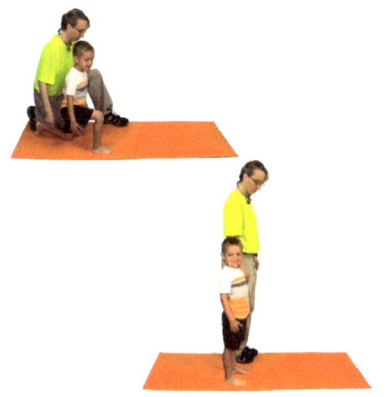

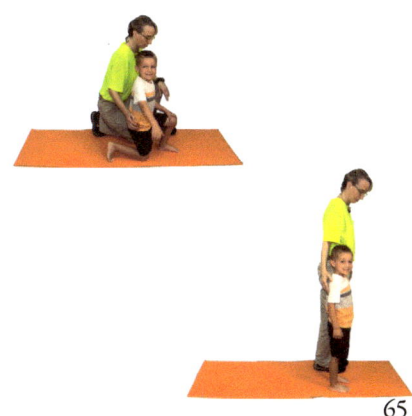

63. ONE LEG SIT TO STAND

I always start with a relatively high seat and then work lower. This activity is so hard. Just an inch higher or lower makes a significant difference in the difficulty level. This exercise is a "go-to" for my more capable clients with hemiplegia or significant one-sided weakness.

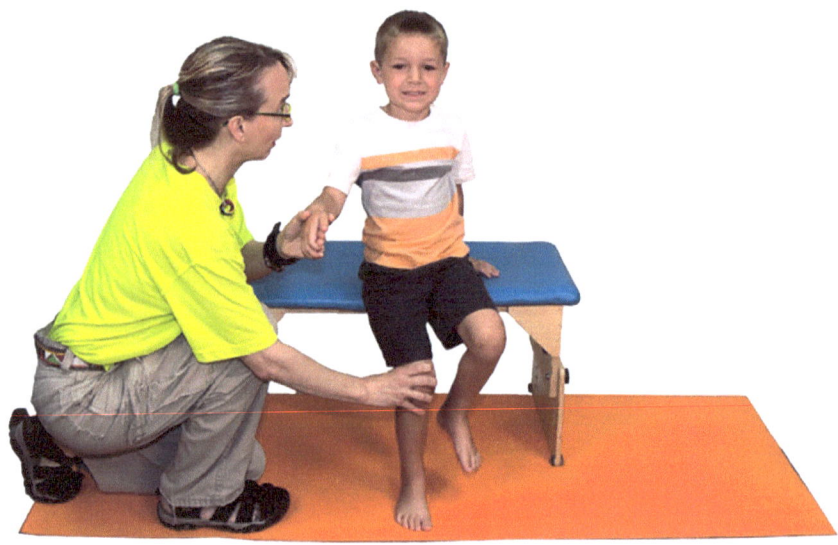

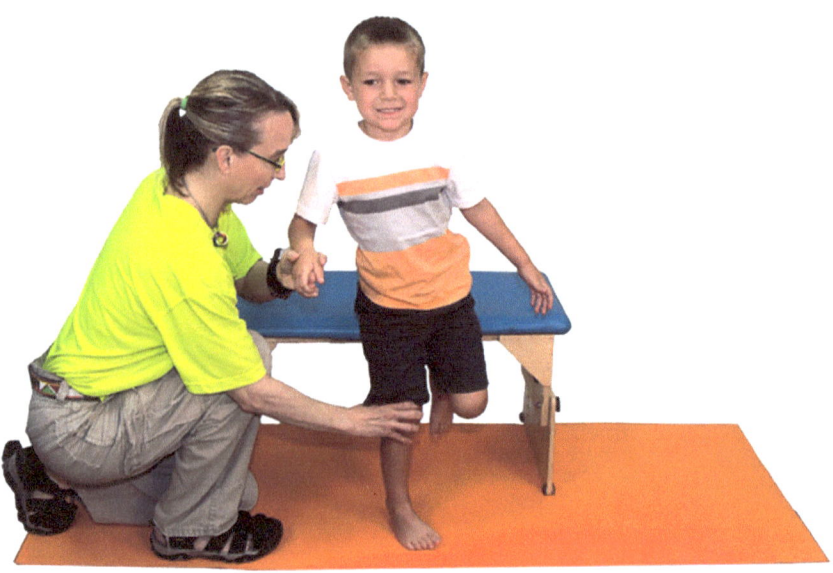

PEDIATRIC PHYSICAL THERAPY STRENGTHENING EXERCISES FOR THE KNEES

64. SQUAT JUMPS

Very fatigue-inducing activity, but my clients don't seem to mind. Often kids don't go into a full squat before the jump. I either verbally cue, "All the way down." or assist at the hips to go all the way down. I do this exercise with the child when I can so we can have all the "fun" together. I have a few children who are unable to assume a full squat, so I will either let them sit on a low bench like a four-inch (10 cm) bench to be able to jump up from or I let them hold onto grips on a wall and jump from a squat with support.

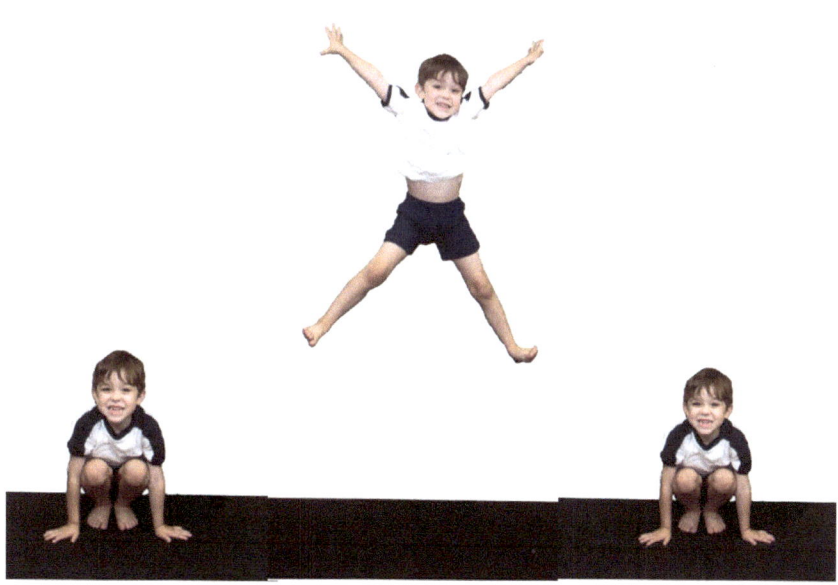

65. BURPEES

I have never known a client who liked burpees. So choose this exercise carefully. This seems to work best for the "hard core" client, specifically the ones who are motivated to excel at a sport. Personally, I like competition for motivation. I challenge my client to a competition of who can do the most repetitions in 30 seconds. I set the timer and have the parent count for the child. I count for myself, and we are off. I almost always get beat. If you want to add an additional challenge to this already difficult task, set a metronome beat to pace a client. See how long you and/or your client can keep pace.

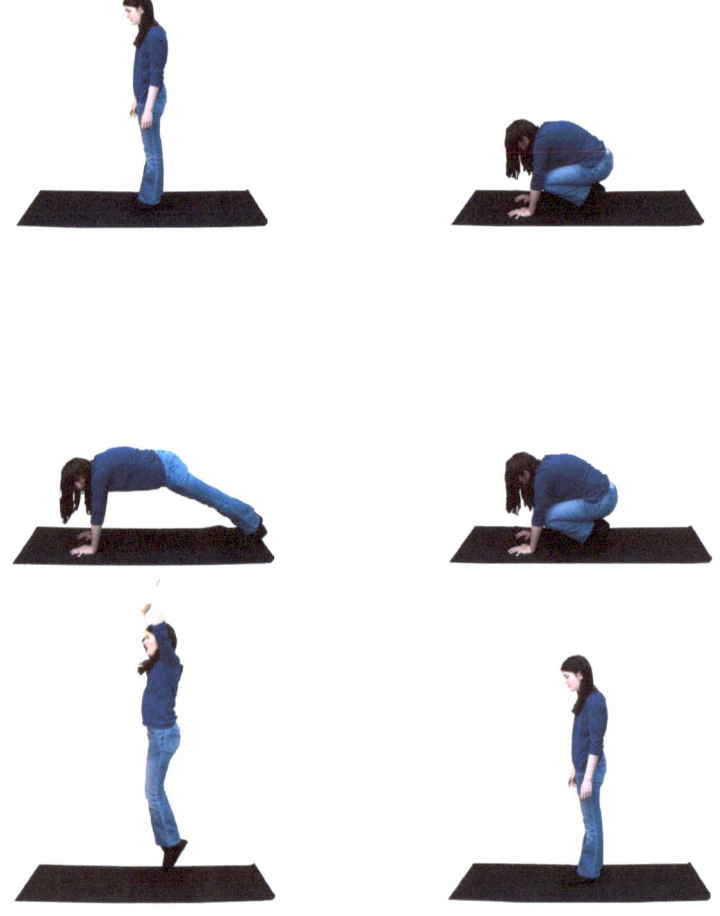

PEDIATRIC PHYSICAL THERAPY STRENGTHENING EXERCISES FOR THE KNEES

II. KNEE FLEXION

THE KNEE FLEXORS MAKE THE angle between the femur and tibia get smaller, and the ankle moves closer to the buttock. This movement is in the sagittal plane. The knee flexors are important for everyday movements like walking and running. Weakness or tightness in the hip flexors will affect gait, sitting and standing posture. As physical therapists we often address spasticity in the hamstrings. A spastic muscle is a weak muscle. Strengthen knee flexors to gain more voluntary control of the knee flexors. This chapter includes a wide variety of exercises to improve knee flexor strength.

* * *

1. HIP/KNEE FLEXION SUPINE ON THE BALL

Yes, I use this activity for knee flexion or knee extension. This exercise uses gravity to magnify small hip and knee movements. I take clients through the movement so that they can get the feel of the motion. Often the client will be motivated by the action and want to repeat it. I have used this exercise with clients with very significant involvement successfully. If you're going to make it harder, hang the client further off the back of the ball to start. If you want to make it easier, put her more on top of the ball, so she doesn't have to fight gravity as hard.

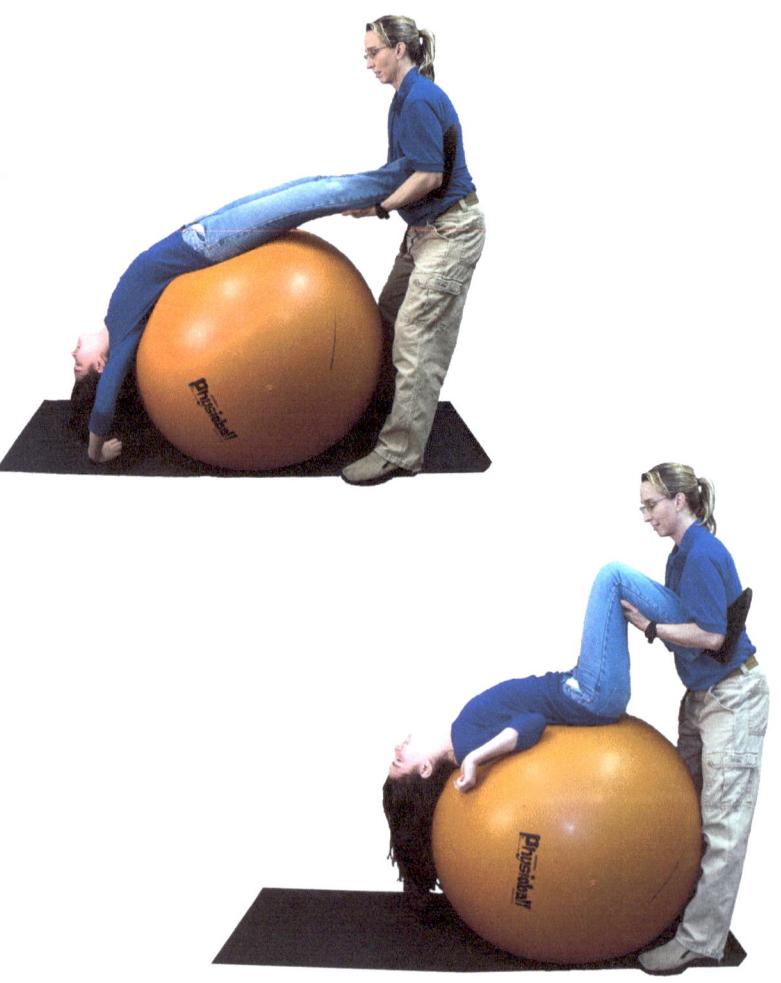

2. SUPINE BICYCLE

This exercise works bilateral alternating hip and knee flexion and extension. You can choose to resist only the flexion component or both the flexion and extension components. The elastic band resistance option is definitely for a higher functioning and cooperative client. I usually perform this activity with manual resistance/assistance. If alternating movements are too hard, you can always revert to symmetrical flexion and extension of the legs.

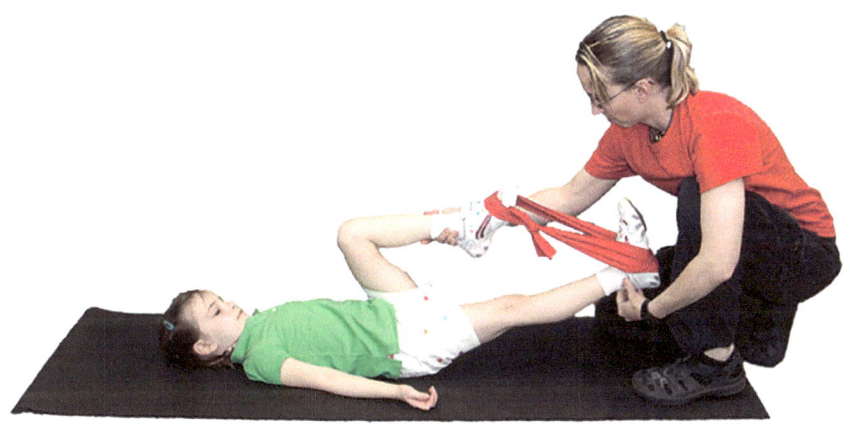

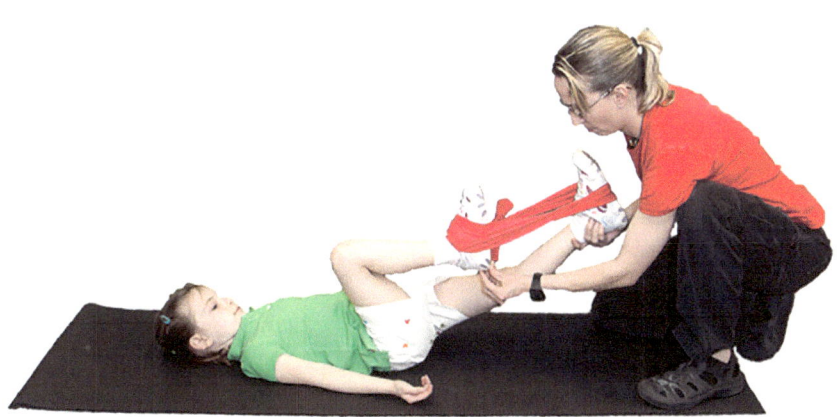

3. BILATERAL KNEE/HIP EXTENSION WITH A SCOOTERBOARD

This exercise is the classic heel slide with a scooterboard flare. Many of my clients with diplegic cerebral palsy are weak in their hamstrings or have spasticity in their hamstrings. I use the scooterboard here to minimize the resistance from the heel sliding along the yoga mat to allow success. If I was worried about the height differential in the way I set up this exercise, I could place my client (and not the scooterboard) on a double-folded exercise mat to even them out. Then the scooterboard and my client on would be more level. I can have the client pull in the scooterboard with one or two feet. To increase the resistance, I put the scooterboard on the carpet as opposed to smooth flooring. I could also add weights to the scooterboard.

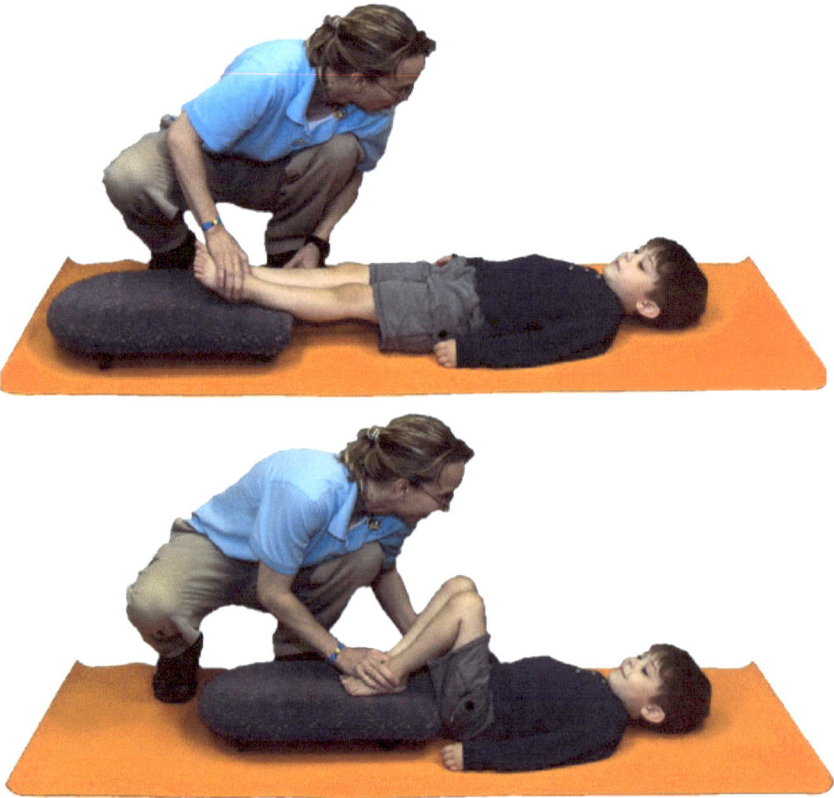

4. SUPINE ELASTIC BAND KNEE FLEXION

This one always seems tricky to me to get the angle of the theratubing right so that it resists knee flexion but doesn't slide right off the heel. Theraband provides more surface area, so it might be a better choice. Different resistance levels are, of course, available in theraband and theratubing.

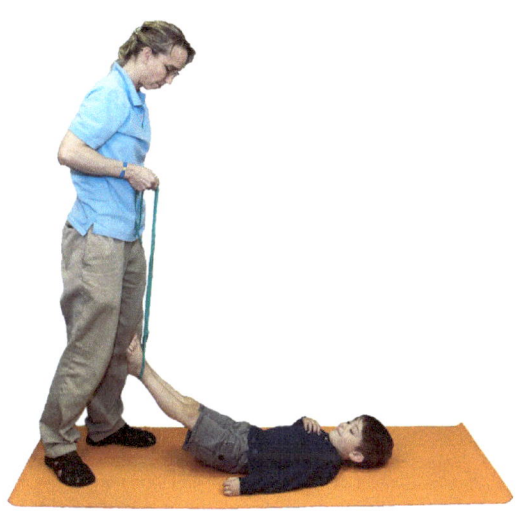

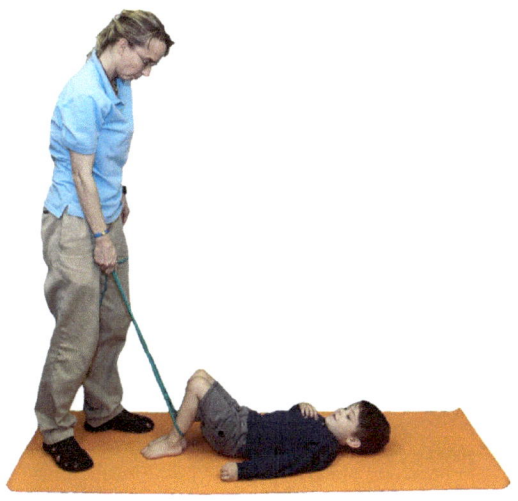

5. ONE LEG BRIDGING

Yes, I know this is a classic hip extension exercise; however, when you lift one leg in a bridge position, the hamstrings work hard to hold the position.

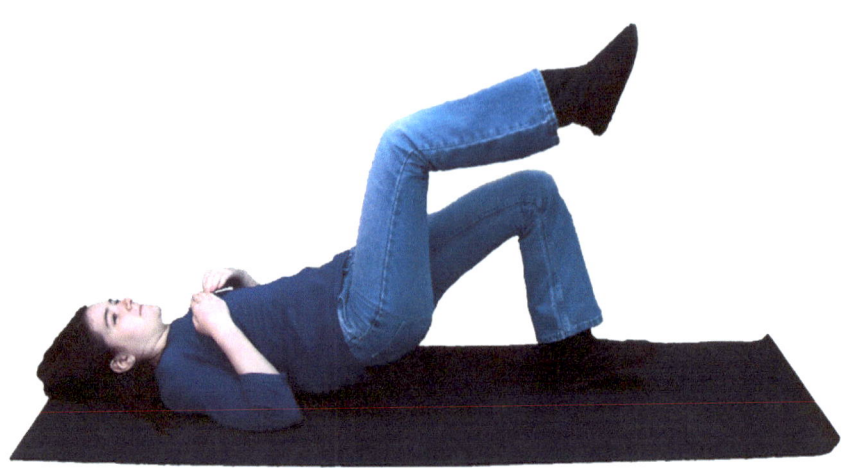

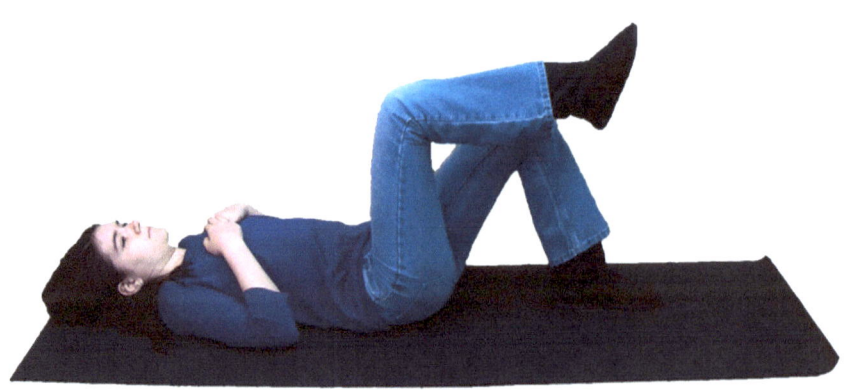

PEDIATRIC PHYSICAL THERAPY STRENGTHENING EXERCISES FOR THE KNEES

6. HIP EXTENSION WITH KNEE FLEXION

Yes, I know this is a another classic hip extension exercise. I believe performing this movement with the knee flexed makes the hamstrings work much harder.

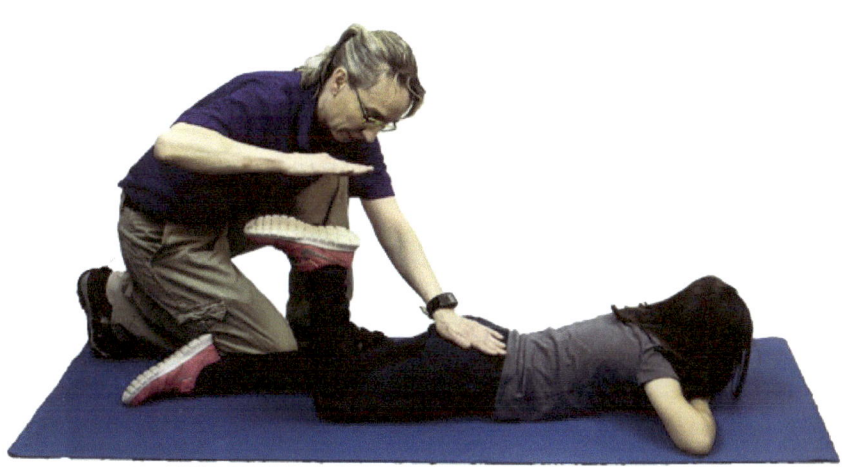

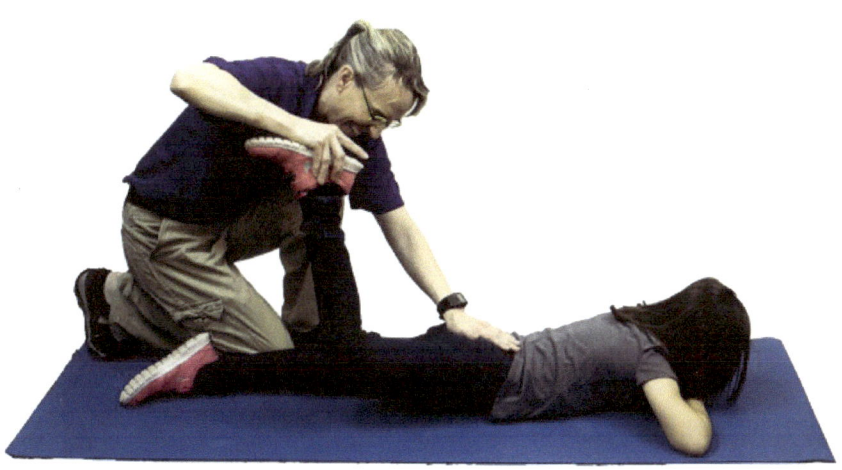

7. HAND TO HEEL TOUCHES

This exercise is fantastic for strengthening the core. But it also targets hamstrings. As you laterally flex, you have to dig your heel in using knee flexion to be able to laterally flex to touch your hand to your heel.

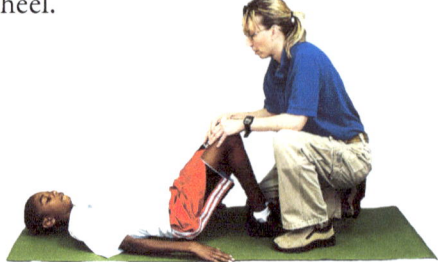

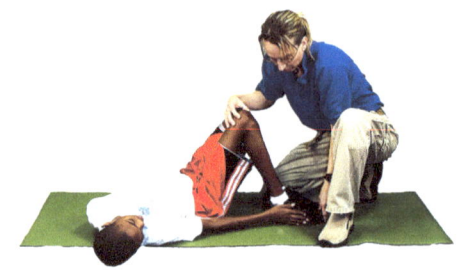

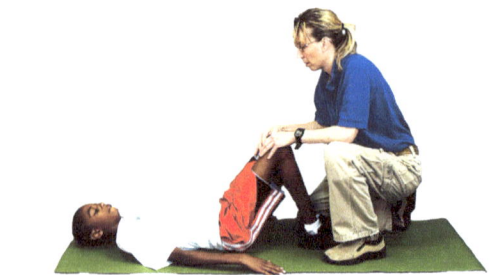

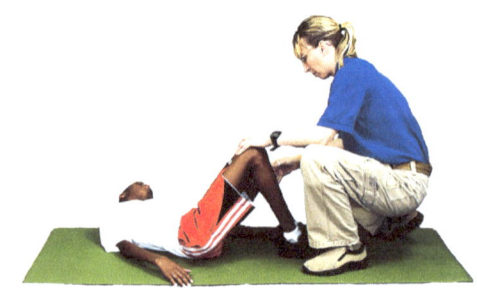

8. TALL KNEEL RESISTED

Holding tall kneeling requires co-contraction at the knee. If given a nudge/push, particularly from posteriorly, hamstrings have to work hard to stabilize and maintain the position.

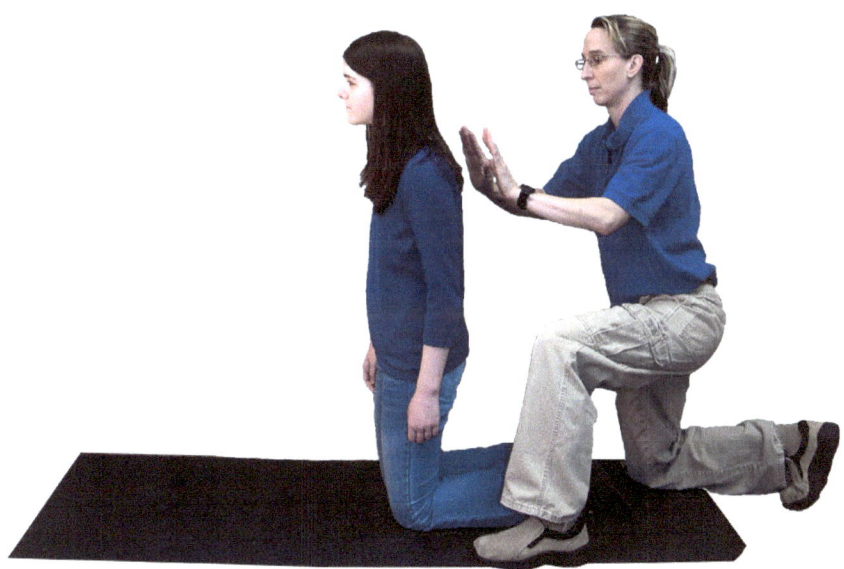

9. TALL KNEEL ON A ROCKERBOARD

The dynamic weight shifting in kneeling requires constant adjustment by the hamstrings. Try side to side and forward/back rocks.

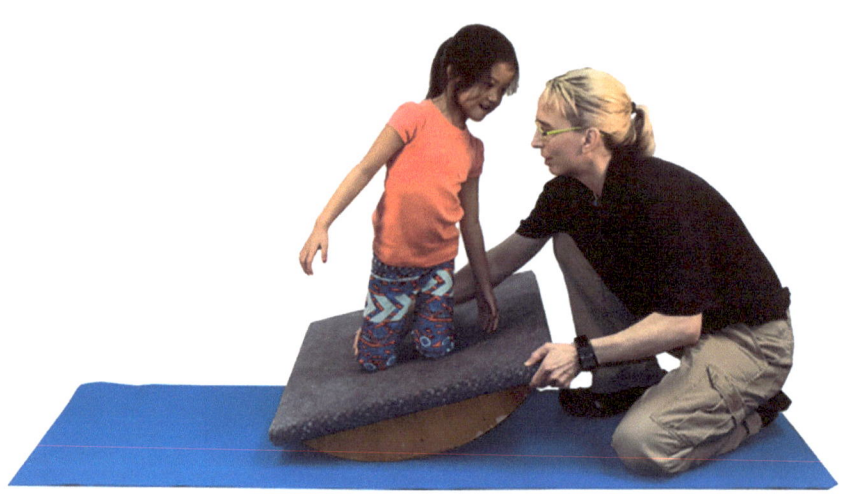

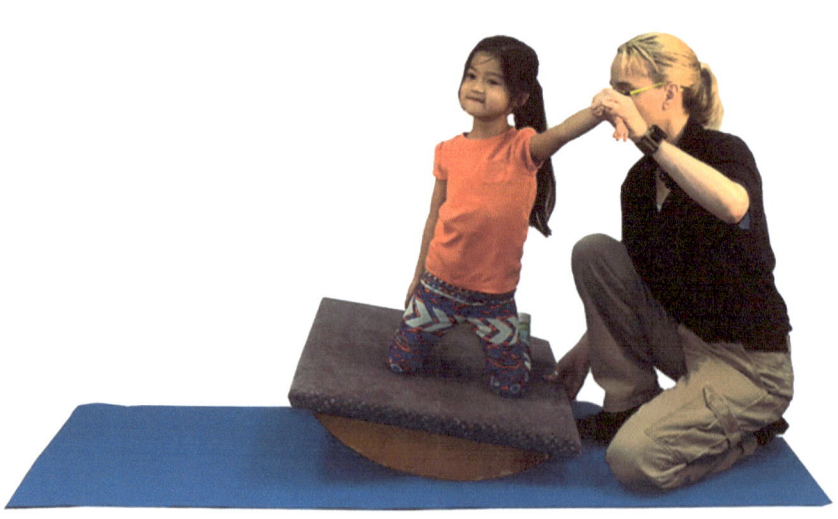

PEDIATRIC PHYSICAL THERAPY STRENGTHENING EXERCISES FOR THE KNEES

10. HALF KNEEL ON ROCKERBOARD

Static positions tend to encourage unengaged muscles. Dynamic movement requires muscle contractions. Start slow and work faster as your child is successful. I tend to impose the motion on the child initially. Then if the child is successful, I see if she can perform the weight shift and rock on her own. Either way, the hamstrings are working hard here.

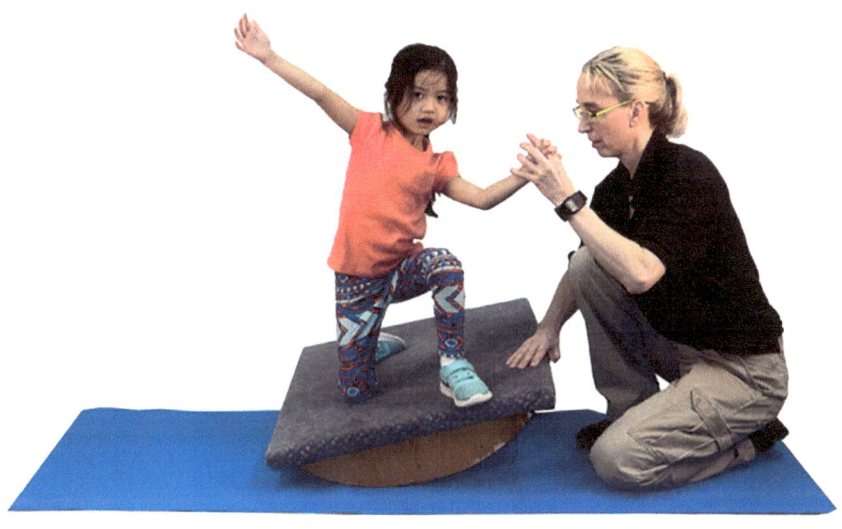

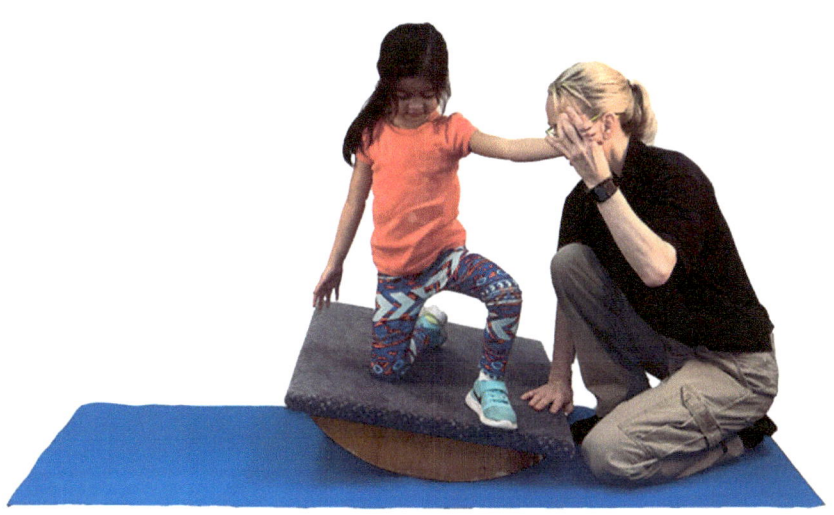

11. PUSH/PULL LEGS WITH PARTNER

This activity is a fun way to work knee flexion and extension control and core strengthening. Why fight it? You both get a workout.

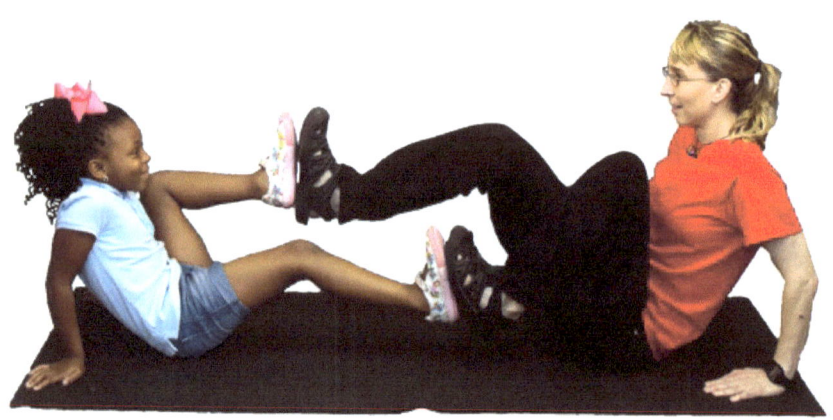

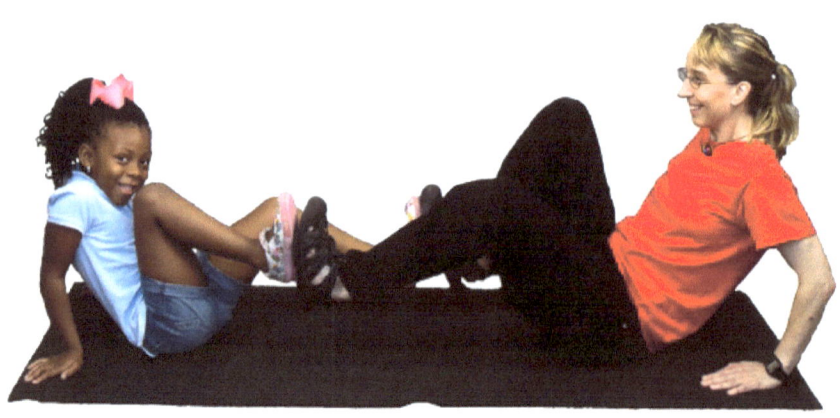

12. SEATED BALL PICK UP

The client picks up the ball. He puts the ball into a hoop or basket that I hold. This motion emphasizes knee flexors and abdominals. Keep the hoop/target higher and closer for more hamstring work.

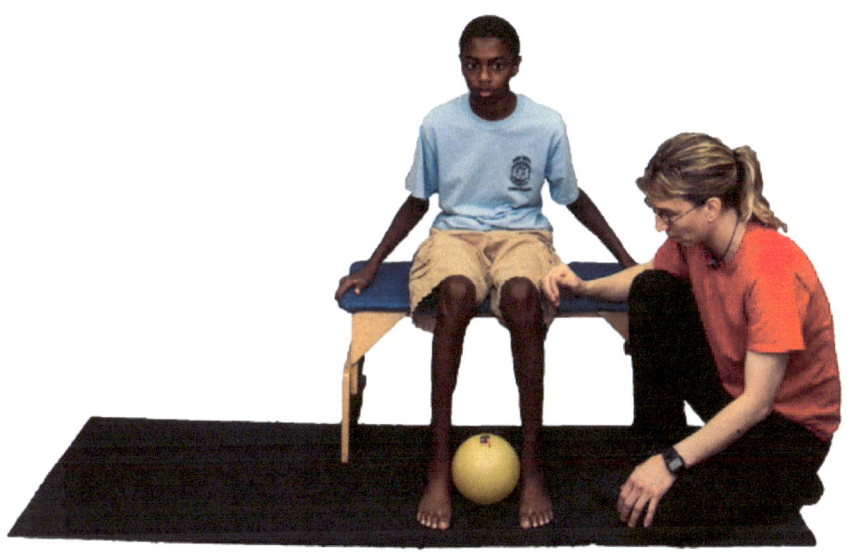

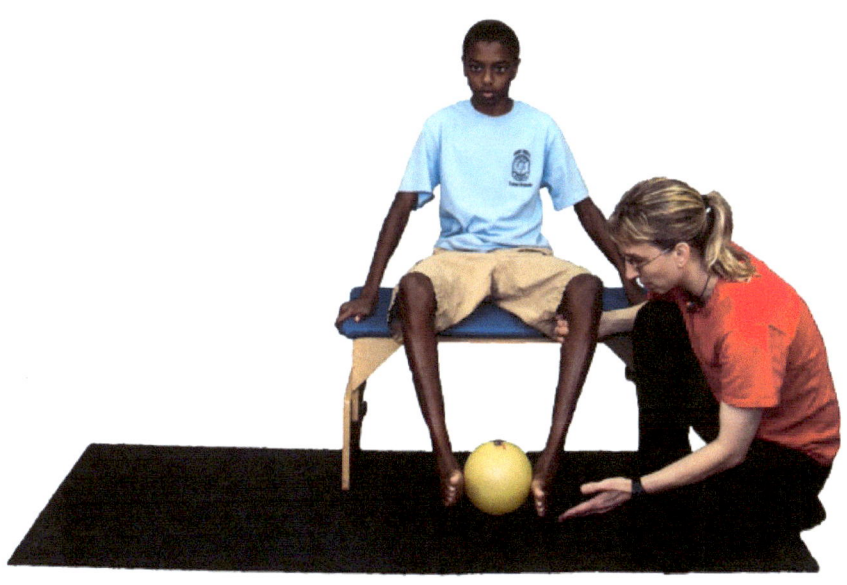

13. PRONE HANG ON THE BOLSTER SWING

I don't know a child who dislikes this activity. I am always amazed at how hard it is for many children to pull in their knee flexors to be able to squeeze the bolster. Once I get a child on the bolster swing, I swing it gently or wildly according to what I think the child can tolerate. I love singing "Engine Engine Number Nine" as I swing the bolster swing, and ask my client to stay on through to the end of the song. Most any childhood song will do. I particularly like the ones used with jump rope games. In the picture, I have the bolster swing hooked up to one attachment point. I prefer to do this activity with the swing set up at two connection points. I set it up with one connection point for the ease of the photo. If the child needs more help, I like to ride on the bolster swing as well, if there is room, just below the child's feet. If I am riding on the bolster swing too, it is easy for me to assist the child to hold on with his legs. If kids don't hold on with their legs, they get thrown off the swing or start rolling off to the side quickly. Be careful with the height of the swing. Most kids fall off. I want the height above a cushioned mat to be safe for a tumble.

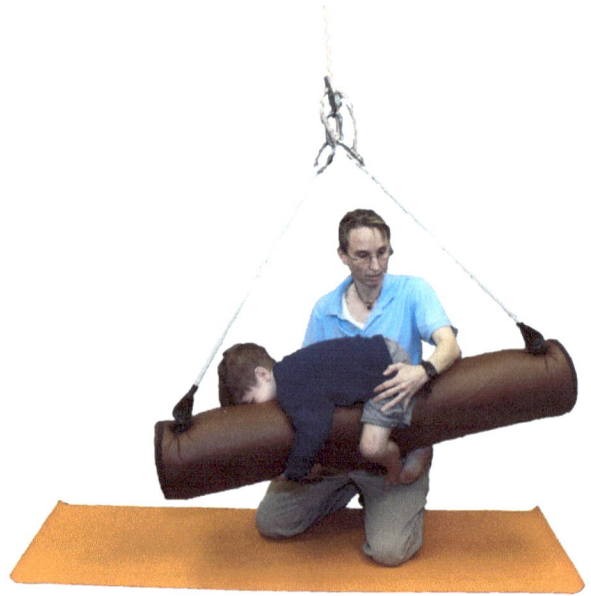

PEDIATRIC PHYSICAL THERAPY STRENGTHENING EXERCISES FOR THE KNEES

14. UPSIDE DOWN ON A BOLSTER SWING

Now the bolster swing is getting fun. A lot of my kids on my caseload are not strong enough to pull off this trick. The child gets on top of the bolster, then he loosens his grip a little and slides to the bottom. This exercise requires a great deal of upper body, hamstring, and adductor strength. To make it really fun, I let a sibling or me take turns with the child. If I am selected, I let the child swing me and try to shake me off. Mayhem and laughter almost always ensue. Just a note, I try to make the floor a safe distance away. You want it to be high enough to get head clearance if he doesn't keep his chin tucked, but low enough that it doesn't hurt to fall off onto a cushioned mat.

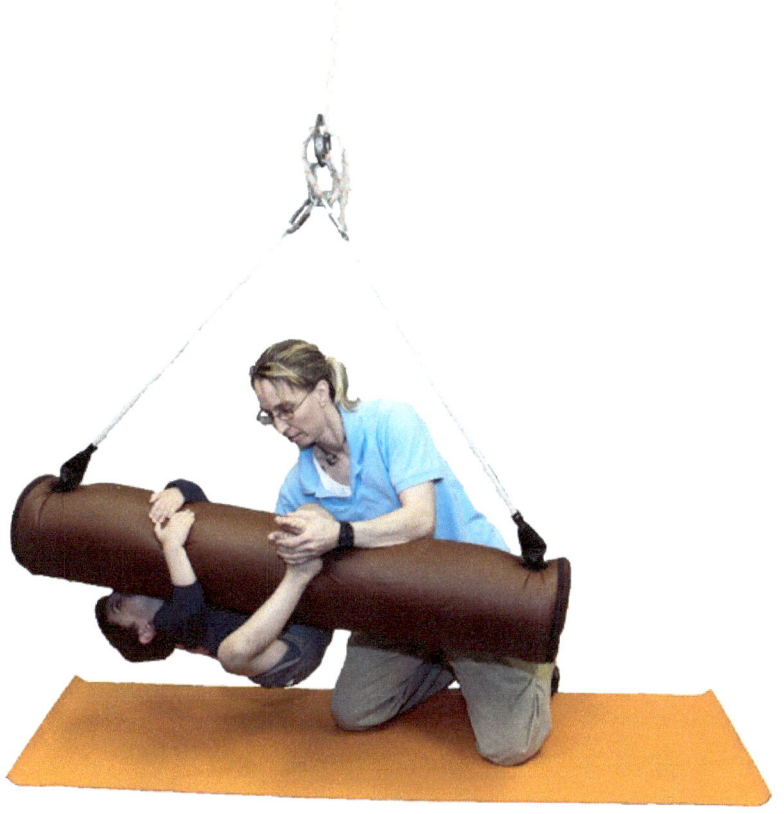

15 UPSIDE DOWN HANG FROM A POLE

Don't let it discourage you if you don't have a bolster swing. Have two people pick up either end of a pole, lifting the child in the middle, and you have almost as much fun. I recommend this over a bean bag or an ottoman. We usually lift and then wiggle or swing a little. Who knew hamstring work could be so much fun.

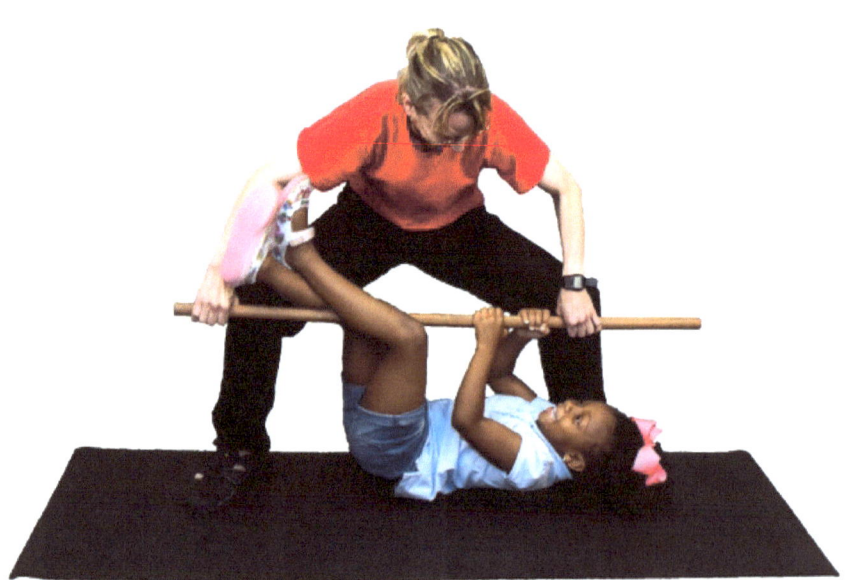

PEDIATRIC PHYSICAL THERAPY STRENGTHENING EXERCISES FOR THE KNEES

16. SITTING ON A BOLSTER SWING

Just sitting and hanging on, especially without upper extremity support, makes kids hold on tightly with their hamstrings. At least some kids do. Some kids let their legs hang limply. Of course, these are the ones who need to work their hamstrings. You may have to teach them how to hold on with their legs.

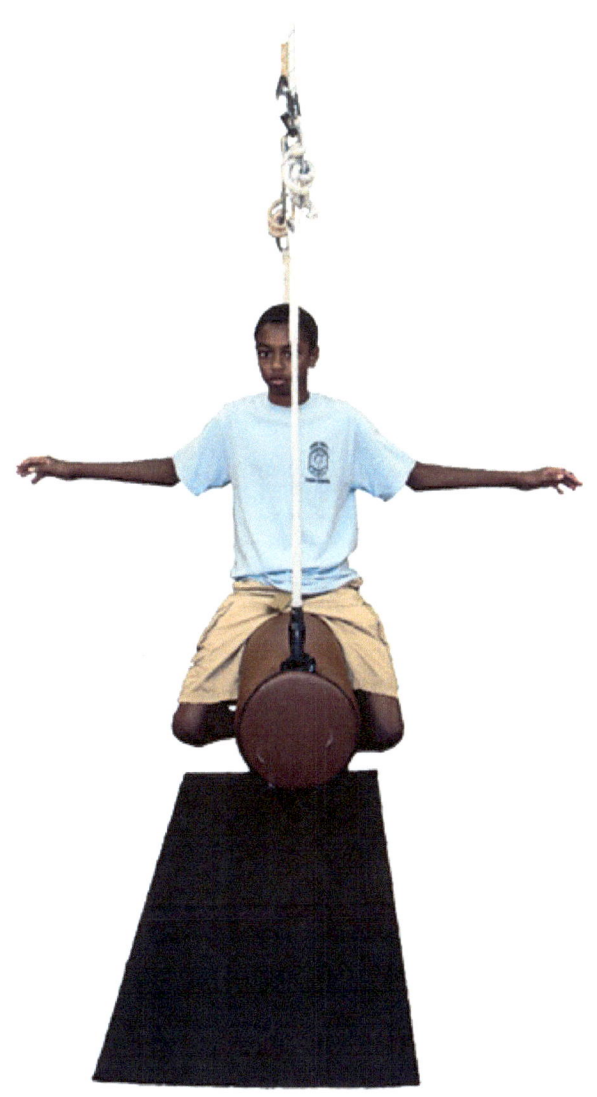

17. SITTING ON A BALL SWING

Don't have a bolster swing. Try tying up a ball in a net swing. Have the child sit on it and hold on. I have so many clients who haven't got a clue how to hold on with their hamstrings. The wider the swing excursion, the more the hamstrings work.

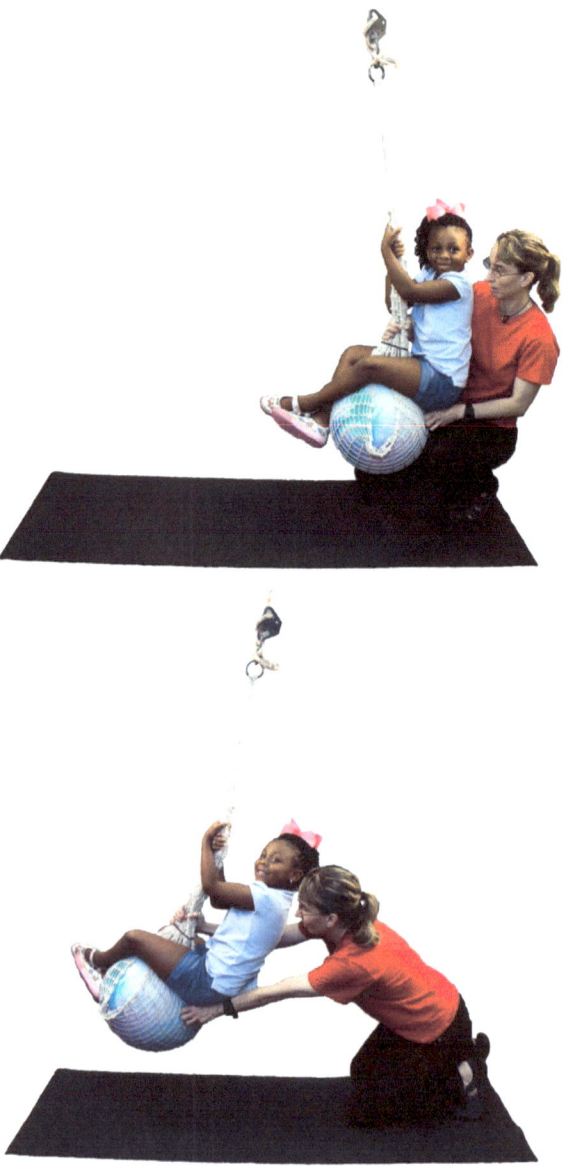

18. LEANED BACK SITTING ON A BALL

Don't have a swing. Try leaning back your client on a ball. Yes, this works abdominals, but clients also tend to recruit their hamstrings to hold on for dear life.

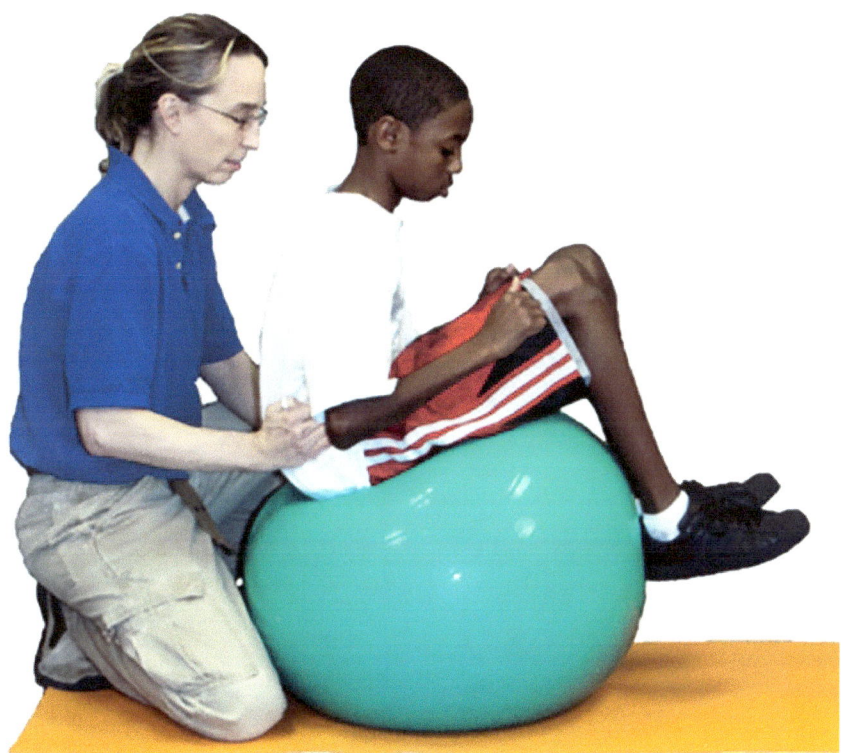

19. SCOOT FORWARD SUPINE

This exercise is deceivingly tough. I had to fake it on the yoga mat. I do this exercise on a smooth floor. I stabilize the child's heels on the floor and ask the child to pull himself toward me with the strength of his hamstrings. To make this a lot easier, you could have the child lying supine on a scooterboard, which would effectively overcome the resistance of the floor.

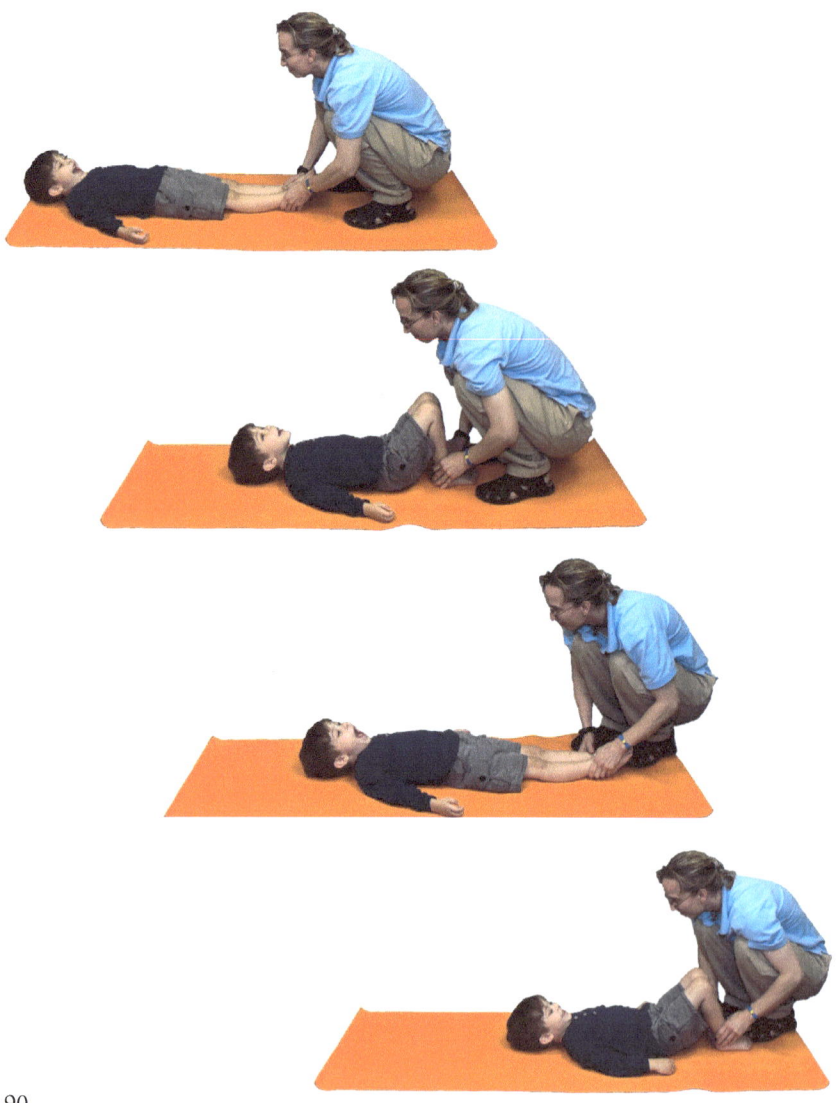

PEDIATRIC PHYSICAL THERAPY STRENGTHENING EXERCISES FOR THE KNEES

20. CRAB WALK

Oh, the dreaded crab walk. I usually get down on the floor and do it too. Why not get a work out as well? If I complain about the exercise, it seems like the kids don't mind so much. To get hamstrings particularly active, I have the child go forward, i.e., feet first. I always emphasize keeping the hips off the ground, with more or less success. I may set up races going down the hall. A child is not so miserable crab walking if she is beating her therapist in a hot race. I have also played soccer in this position with my client.

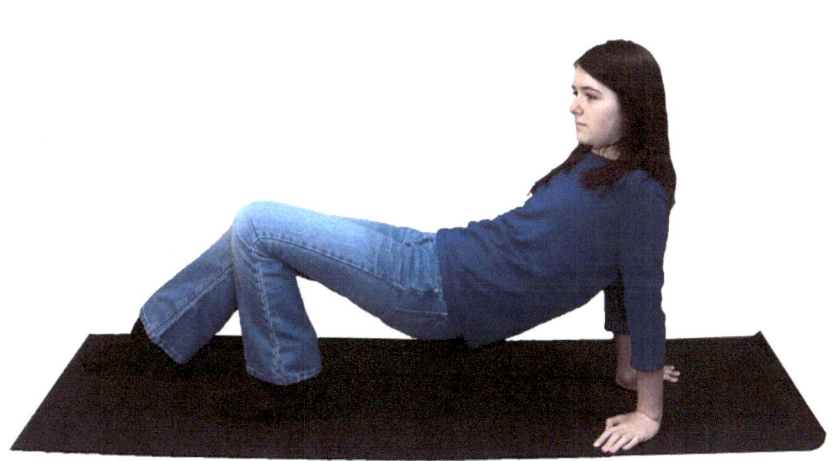

21. PRONE KNEE FLEXION

I perform this activity one leg at a time or bilaterally. I usually give manual resistance, but Velcro ankle weights are an excellent way to objectify the progress. If a child has on orthotic, I will often set the activity up so that the child's feet are hanging off the mat or mat table to be more comfortable. With my clients with diplegic cerebral palsy, they can usually take mild resistance at the beginning of the range, then I switch to no resistance, then as they get close to 90 degrees knee flexion or more, I usually have to assist.

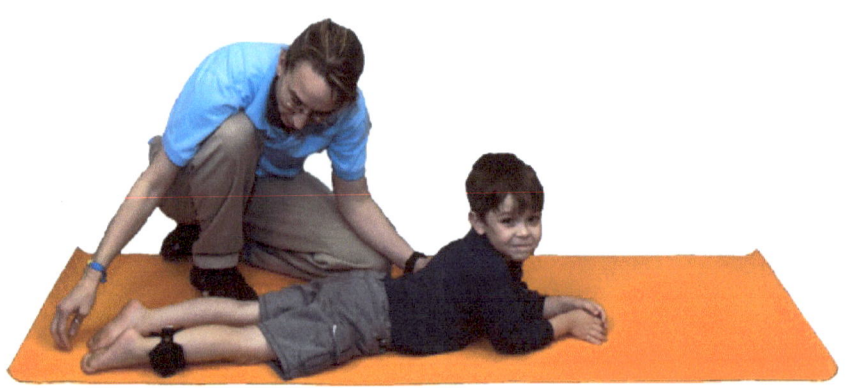

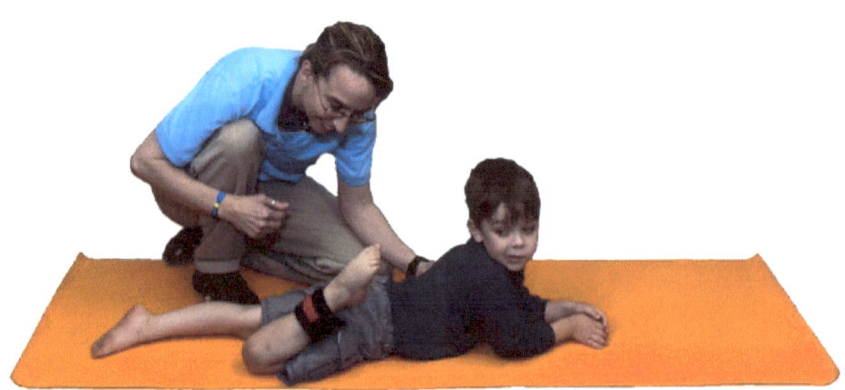

22. HOLD KNEE FLEXION TO RIDE

This activity is surprisingly hard for several clients. To go, the child simply has to maintain knee flexion while she rides on the scooterboard. If she drops her feet, then I stop the ride. Simple but fun and effective. This exercise works the same prone on a platform swing.

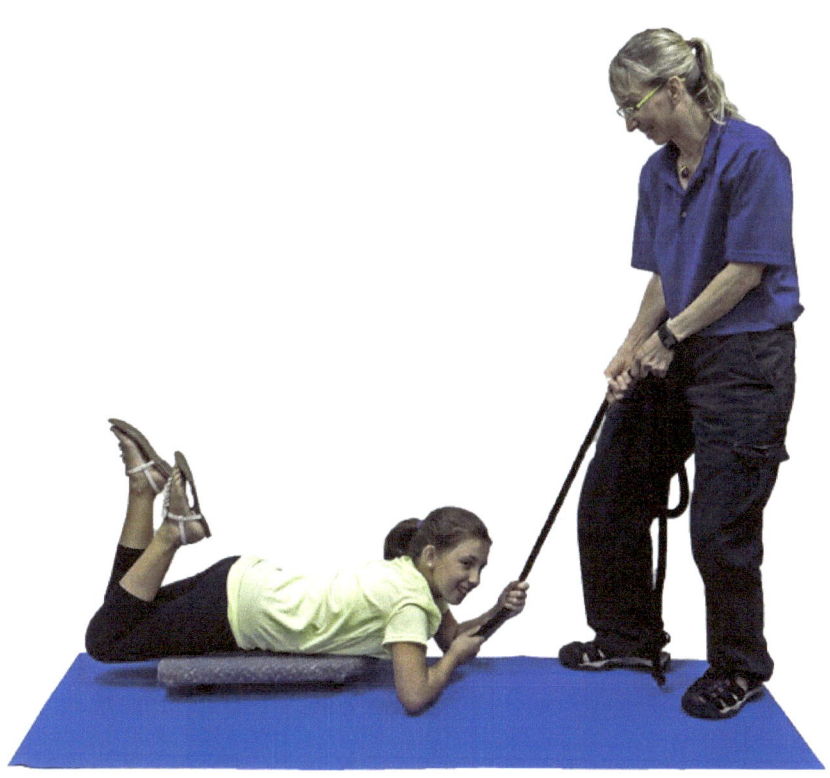

23. PRONE RIDE WITH LEG PULL

Since holding knee flexion is hard for my children with neurological impairment, I made up this game. The child only has to keep his knees flexed to be able to be pulled by his heels. I carefully choose my floor surface. Many of my children with diplegia need to be on the smoother vinyl floors to be able to hold the knee flexion to be able to go. I can pull the stronger ones down the carpeted hallway. I use the acceleration and deceleration of me pulling the child's feet to add to the child's workout. The same game works for a child swinging prone on a platform swing as well.

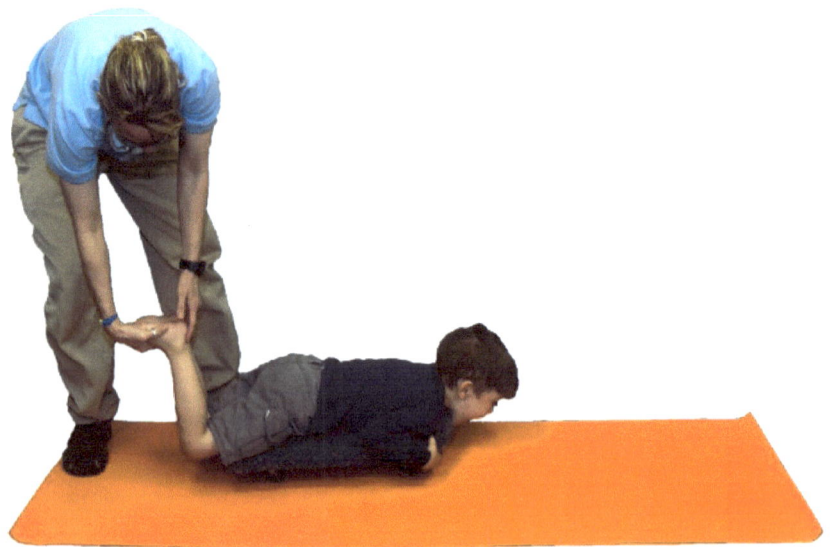

24. SITTING MANUAL RESISTANCE KNEE FLEXION

Any time a boy can knock down a block, he is happy. I vary the manual resistance or assistance as needed according the range. I may add fuel to the fire by saying something like this, "I bet you can't knock down the block by the time I count to 5!" It becomes a "me against them" game. And my goodness, they do like to win. I also perform this exercise eccentrically. I start with the client in knee flexion, and I make the opposite bet. I say something like, "I bet I can get your toes up to my nose before I count to 10!" I pull the leg straight, and the child eccentrically resists. I provide just enough resistance to make sure I lose. The more I protest losing, the more fun this game is.

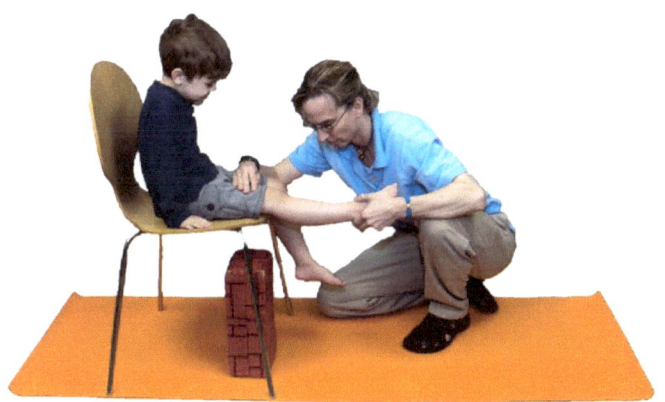

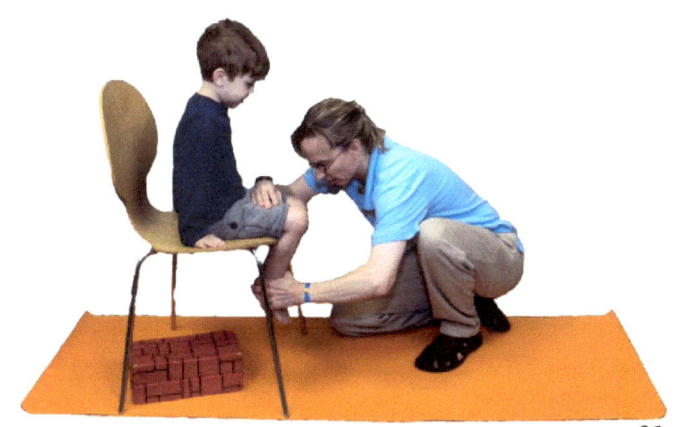

25. NET SWING WITH KNEE FLEXION

Swinging is one of the ways kids love working on knee flexion. Here the child has to keep her knees tightly flexed to be swung. Kids love it!

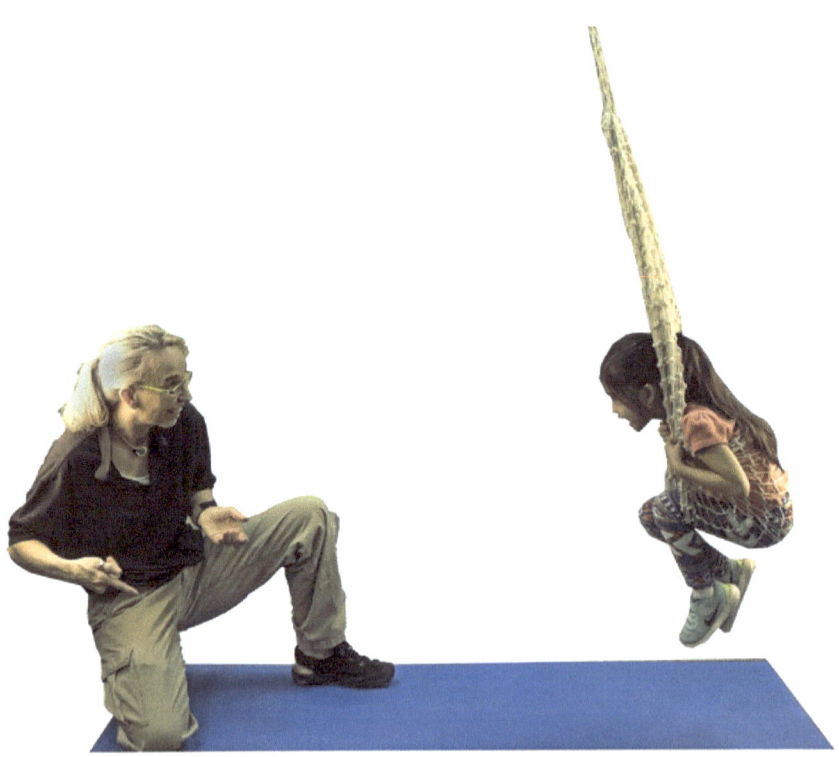

26. TRAPEZE WITH KNEE FLEXION

I place the trapeze bar low enough that knee flexion is required to swing. The hands tend to wear out quickly too, so this is time-limited.

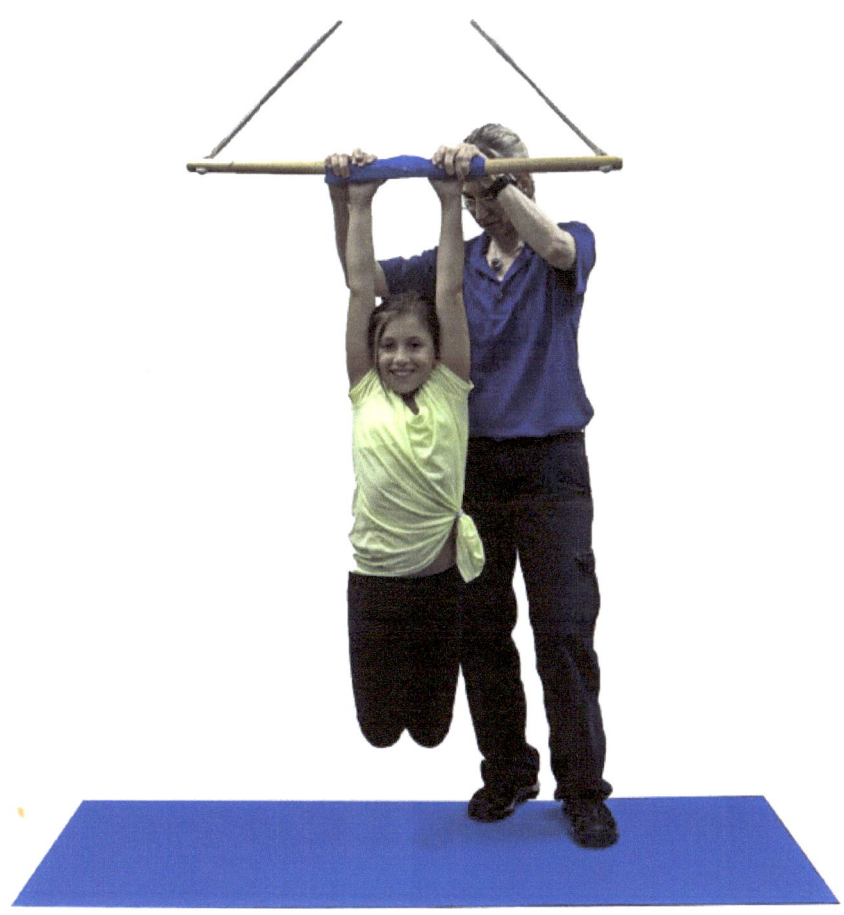

27. SCOOTERBOARD SIT, TWO-LEG PULL

My clients like this knee flexion work the best. I race the child to the other end of the hall at the clinic. I only play this game on smooth floors. We have vinyl tile flooring at the clinic. It would be too hard on carpeting. I have to admit, my hamstrings get tired fast also, but kids love to race and particularly to beat me in a race. The more I complain, the more they like it. When a client is first learning how to self-propel a scooterboard sitting, I stabilize the heels, as seen here.

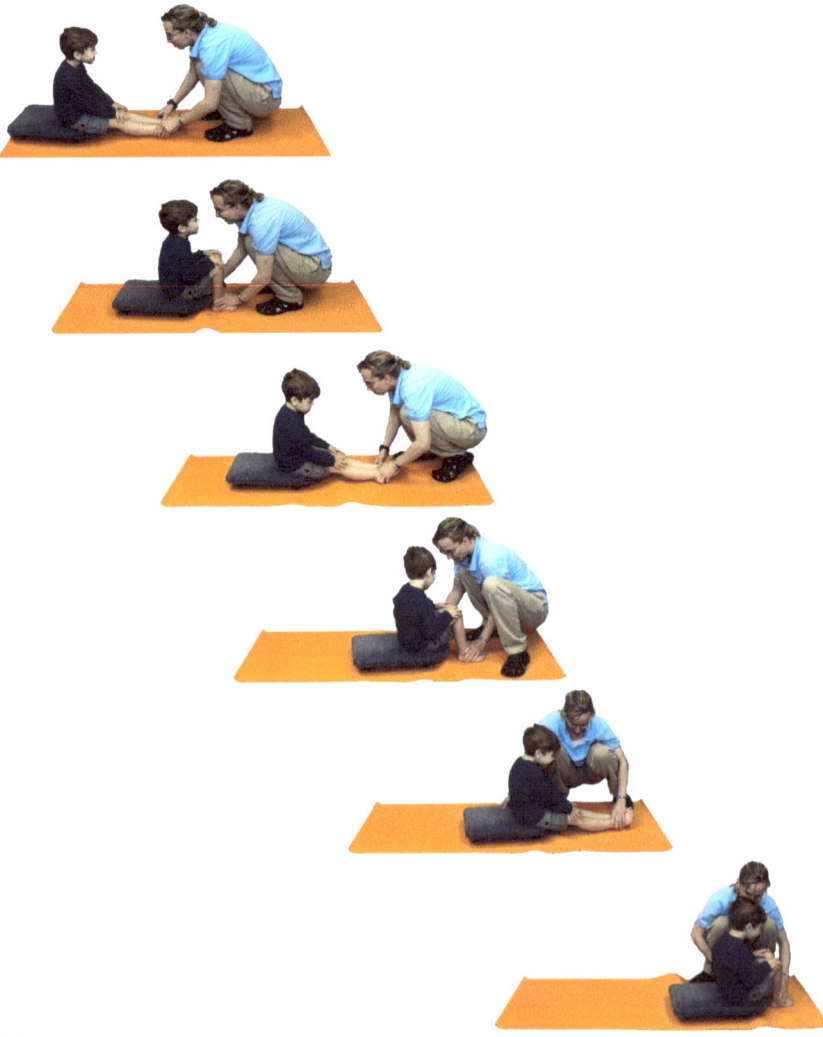

PEDIATRIC PHYSICAL THERAPY STRENGTHENING EXERCISES FOR THE KNEES

28. SCOOTER SIT, ALTERNATE-LEG PROPEL

This exercise is just one step harder than the two-leg propel version. By alternating legs, each leg must pull the weight of the participant. When a client is first learning how to self-propel a scooterboard sitting, I stabilize the heels but not afterward. A rolling desk chair works just as well for this and the previous activity too!

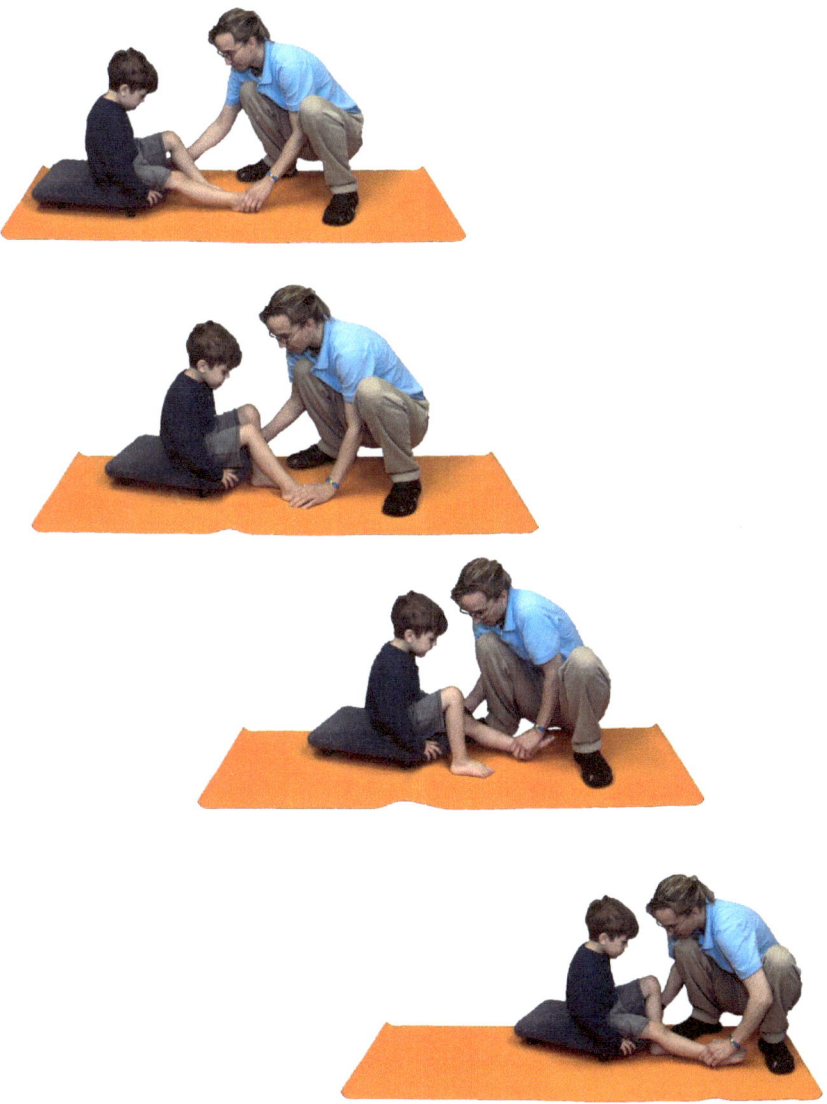

29. SCOOT IN SITTING

I am pretty sure I faked this picture series. I always do this activity on a smooth floor to minimize the resistance. Make sure you stabilize the child's heel enough to have the traction to pull forward. This is very hard work, but not as hard as the supine version of this. Less contact with the floor makes for less friction moving forward.

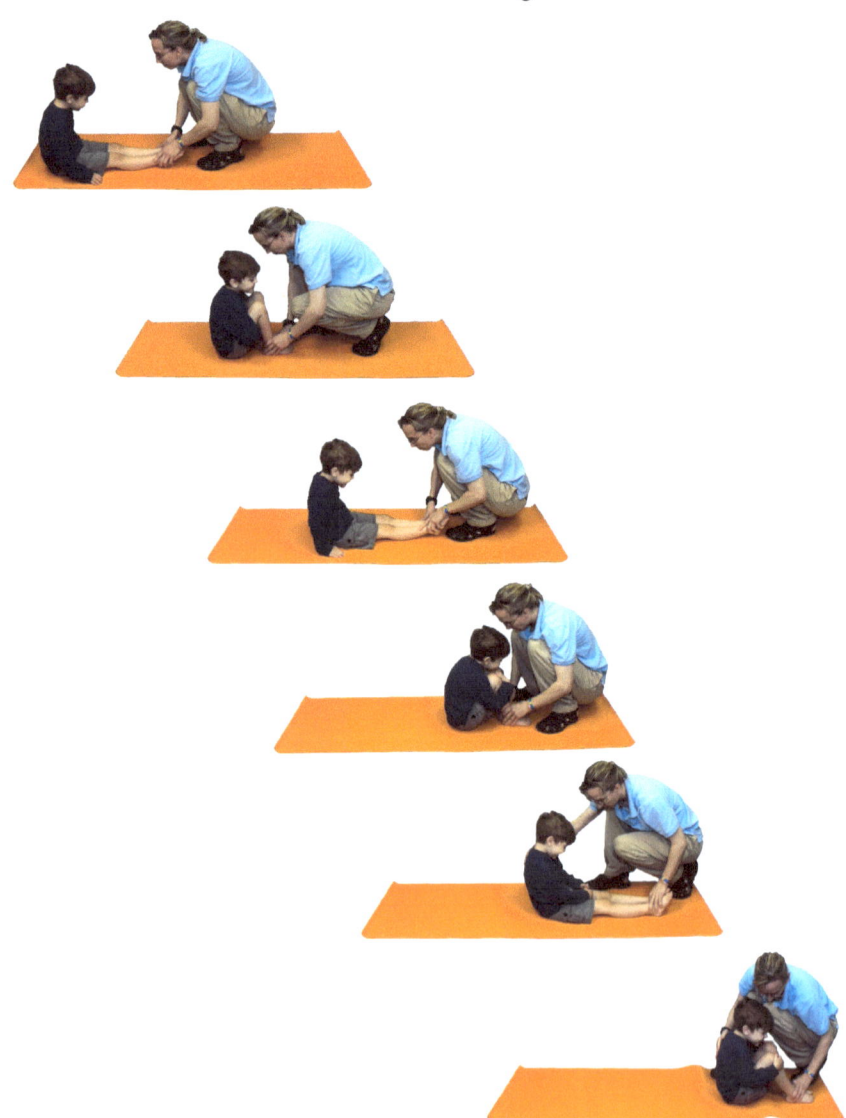

30. SCOOT BACK LYING

Only perform this exercise with children who are really motivated or really love you. No one else. Super hard! You could put the child on a scooterboard to make it easier.

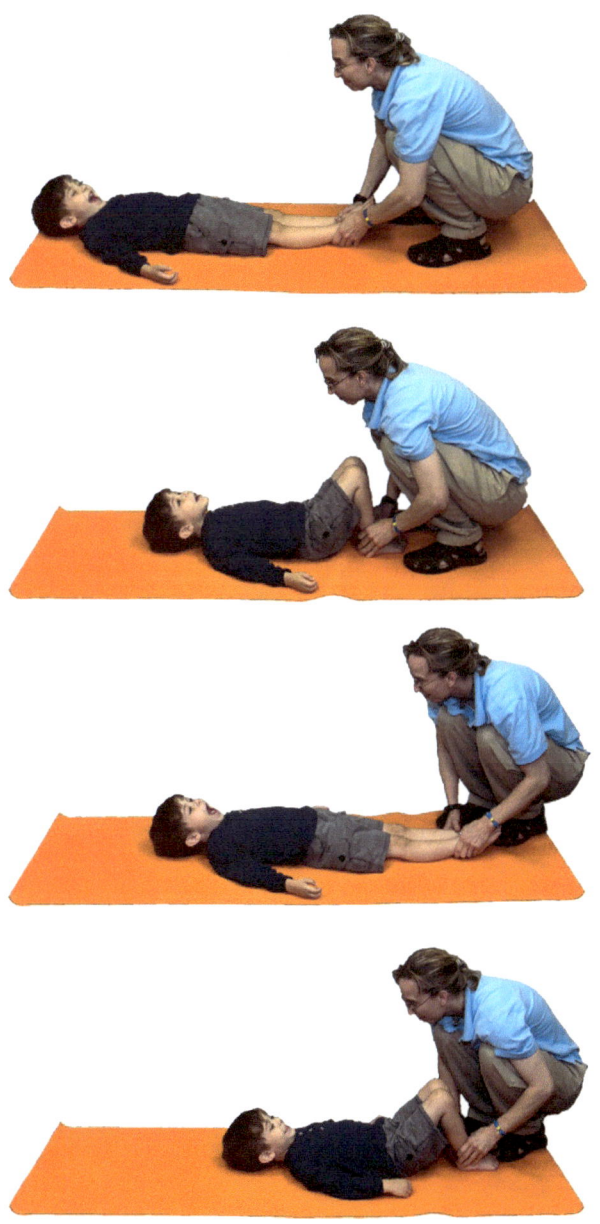

31. STAND AND TOUCH ONE FOOT IN BACK

Often the client requires external support for balance. I typically help the child flex his knee to bring up his foot. I usually provide my hand as a target. I often have to assist at the end range. I see a lot of knee flexion with hip flexion in the child's attempts to do this. Knee flexion with hip extension is much trickier. My model makes it look so easy.

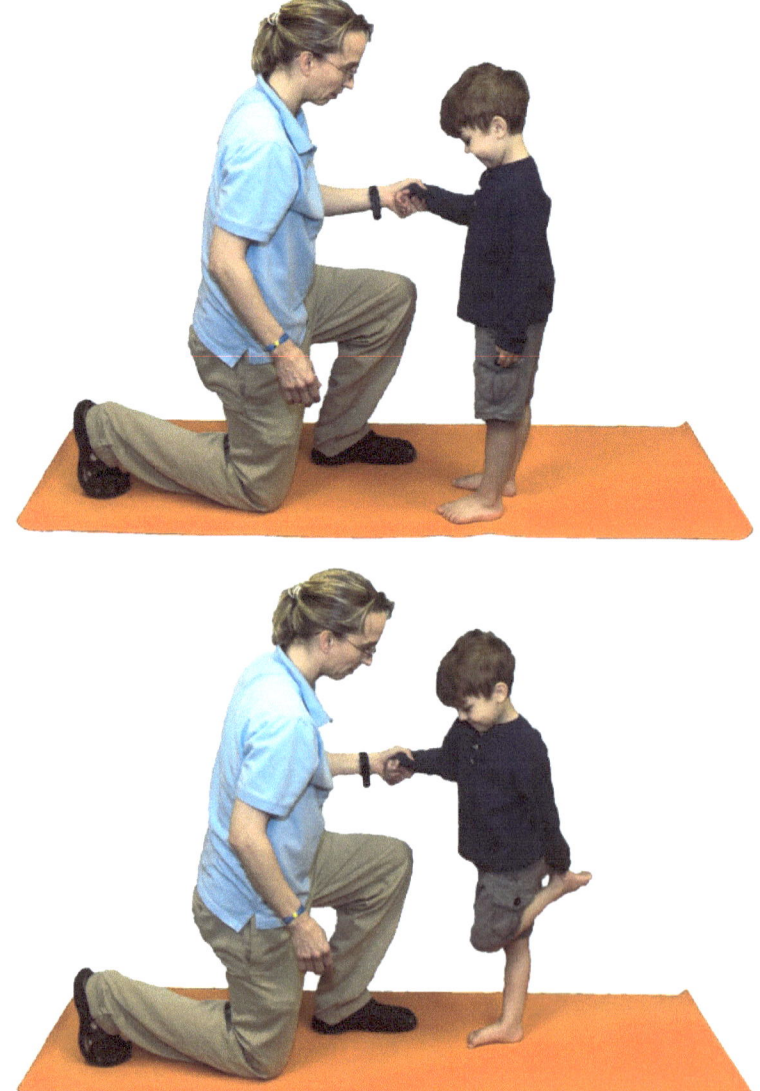

32. STAND AND TOUCH ONE FOOT IN FRONT

For some children, I'll put a sticker or a piece of tape on the bottom of their shoe. For others, I just request ten on each side. I have performed this activity sitting or standing. I think either work hamstrings well.

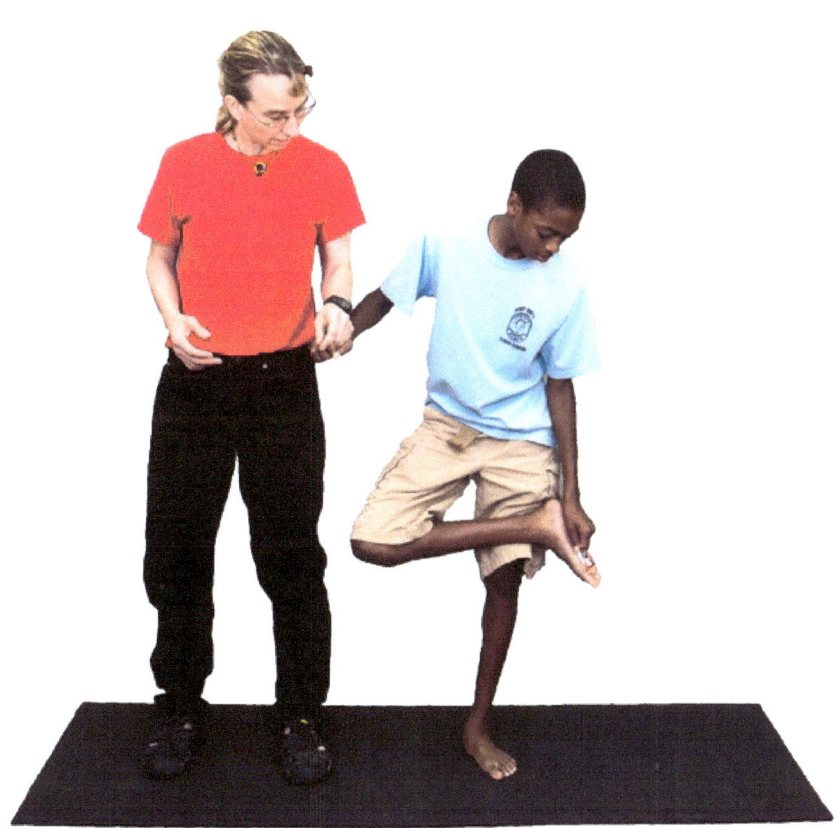

33. JUMP GRABBING HEELS IN BACK

Okay, full disclosure here; these pictures were digitally modified. I love this jump for teaching clients who are ready for the challenge of activating hamstrings quickly in a coordinated move. At first I just try to have the child jump and flex his legs. For many clients, this requires two hands held or supported on a railing. They work to get knee flexion progressively higher. Then I ask the child just to touch one foot and then both. The trampoline is always easier than the floor. I remember when this was on the Bruininks-Oseretsky Test of Motor Proficiency, First Edition. Whew, I was happy when the second edition was released. This jump was no longer on the test.

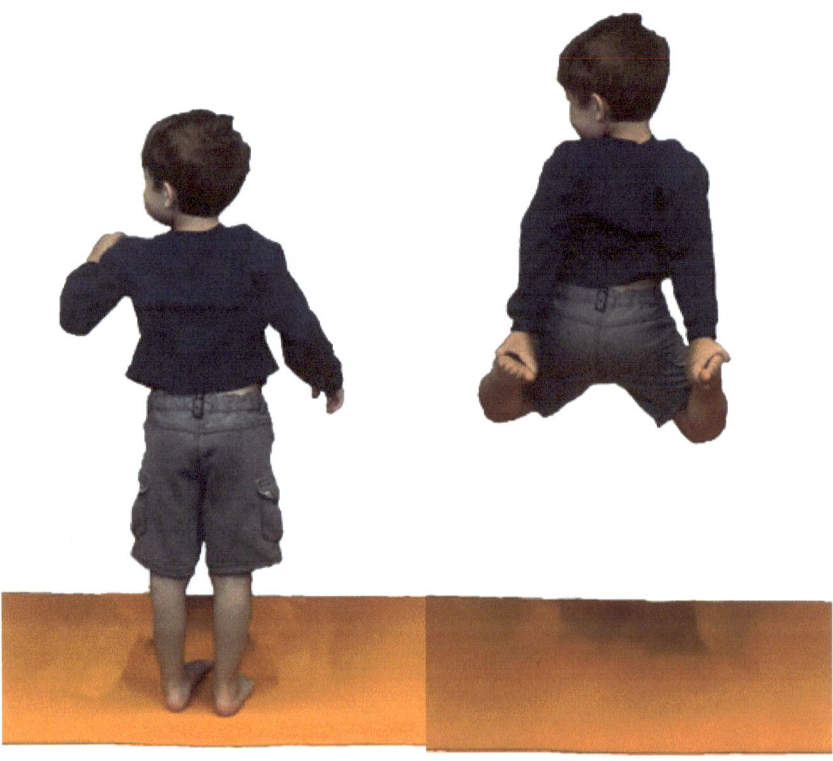

34. HIP EXTENSION PRONE WITH KNEE EXTENSION

When you can do these two jumps, you have mastered your hamstrings speed and control. I let clients start by jumping up and bringing up knees. Next, I have clients jump, tuck, and touch hands to knees. Then I have them jump and grab their knees, bringing knees to chest.

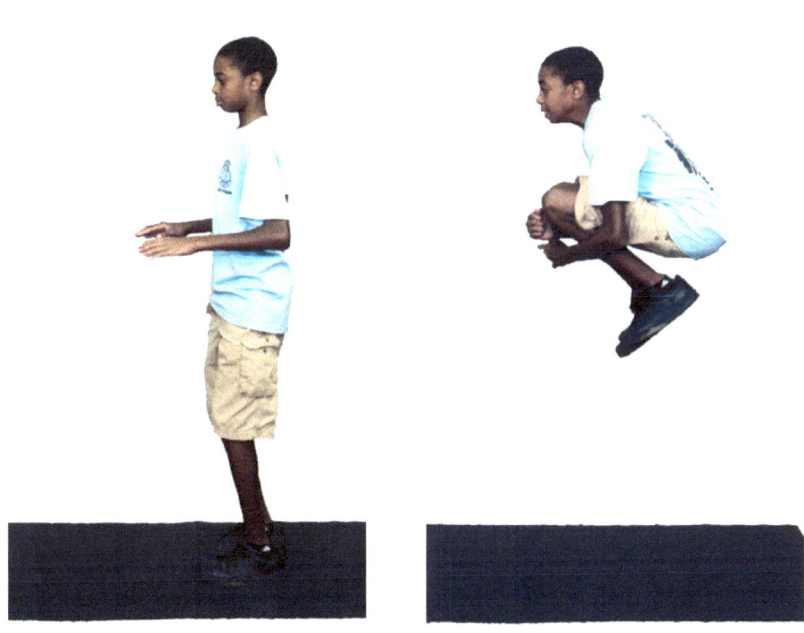

| AMY E. STURKEY, PT

ABOUT THE AUTHOR

AMY STURKEY IS AN OUTPATIENT pediatric physical therapist in Charlotte, NC. Amy won Outstanding PT for North Carolina for 2016. Amy met an adorable boy with cerebral palsy and his family on a safari in Kenya. As she tried to help them, she realized that little information was available to help train pediatric therapists and to educate children and families about common childhood conditions and treatment options. After 30+ years of clinical experience, she decided she had information to share. Amy co-founded Gotcha Apps to produce educational products for pediatric therapists and their clients. She created an instructional Facebook page, a website, and a YouTube channel. Through these platforms, she releases weekly videos to instruct therapists and families of children with physical challenges.

OTHER OFFERINGS BY THE AUTHOR

A is for Autism: A Child's View
D is for Down Syndrome: A Child's View
C is For Cerebral Palsy: A Child's View
Pediatric Physical Therapy Strengthening Exercises for the Hips

Coming Soon:
A is for ADHD: A Child's View

Blog:
www.PediatricPTexercises.com

YouTube Channel:
Pediatric Physical Therapy Exercises

Facebook page:
Pediatric Physical Therapy Exercises

Instagram page:
Pediatric PT Exercises

Pinterest page:
amysturkey/pediatric-physical-therapy